CATARACT: WHAT YOU N

MARK WATTS is a consultant at Arrowe Park Hospital, Wirral many information products for patients, including 'Your Cataract Operation', a booklet produced for his own patients. He has written over thirty papers in the medical press, as well as a textbook on eye disease.

Overcoming Common Problems Series

Selected titles
A full list of titles is available from Sheldon Press,
36 Causton Street, London SW1P 4ST, and on our website at
www.sheldonpress.co.uk

Assertiveness: Step by Step
Dr Windy Dryden and Daniel Constantinou

Body Language at Work
Mary Hartley

The Cancer Guide for Men
Helen Beare and Neil Priddy

The Candida Diet Book
Karen Brody

The Chronic Fatigue Healing Diet
Christine Craggs-Hinton

Cider Vinegar
Margaret Hills

Comfort for Depression
Janet Horwood

Confidence Works
Gladeana McMahon

Coping Successfully with Hay Fever
Dr Robert Youngson

Coping Successfully with Pain
Neville Shone

Coping Successfully with Panic Attacks
Shirley Trickett

Coping Successfully with Prostate Cancer
Dr Tom Smith

Coping Successfully with Prostate Problems
Rosy Reynolds

Coping Successfully with RSI
Maggie Black and Penny Gray

Coping Successfully with Your Hiatus Hernia
Dr Tom Smith

Coping with Alopecia
Dr Nigel Hunt and Dr Sue McHale

Coping with Anxiety and Depression
Shirley Trickett

Coping with Blushing
Dr Robert Edelmann

Coping with Bronchitis and Emphysema
Dr Tom Smith

Coping with Candida
Shirley Trickett

Coping with Childhood Asthma
Jill Eckersley

Coping with Chronic Fatigue
Trudie Chalder

Coping with Coeliac Disease
Karen Brody

Coping with Cystitis
Caroline Clayton

Coping with Depression and Elation
Dr Patrick McKeon

Coping with Down's Syndrome
Fiona Marshall

Coping with Dyspraxia
Jill Eckersley

Coping with Eczema
Dr Robert Youngson

Coping with Endometriosis
Jo Mears

Coping with Epilepsy
Fiona Marshall and
Dr Pamela Crawford

Coping with Fibroids
Mary-Claire Mason

Coping with Gallstones
Dr Joan Gomez

Coping with Gout
Christine Craggs-Hinton

Coping with a Hernia
Dr David Delvin

Coping with Incontinence
Dr Joan Gomez

Coping with Long-Term Illness
Barbara Baker

Coping with the Menopause
Janet Horwood

Coping with a Mid-life Crisis
Derek Milne

Coping with Polycystic Ovary Syndrome
Christine Craggs-Hinton

Coping with Psoriasis
Professor Ronald Marks

Overcoming Common Problems Series

Coping with SAD
Fiona Marshall and Peter Cheevers

Coping with Snoring and Sleep Apnoea
Jill Eckersley

Coping with Stomach Ulcers
Dr Tom Smith

Coping with Strokes
Dr Tom Smith

Coping with Suicide
Maggie Helen

Coping with Teenagers
Sarah Lawson

Coping with Thyroid Problems
Dr Joan Gomez

Curing Arthritis – The Drug-Free Way
Margaret Hills

Curing Arthritis – More Ways to a Drug-Free Life
Margaret Hills

Curing Arthritis Diet Book
Margaret Hills

Curing Arthritis Exercise Book
Margaret Hills and Janet Horwood

Cystic Fibrosis – A Family Affair
Jane Chumbley

Depression at Work
Vicky Maud

Depressive Illness
Dr Tim Cantopher

Effortless Exercise
Dr Caroline Shreeve

Fertility
Julie Reid

The Fibromyalgia Healing Diet
Christine Craggs-Hinton

Getting a Good Night's Sleep
Fiona Johnston

The Good Stress Guide
Mary Hartley

Heal the Hurt: How to Forgive and Move On
Dr Ann Macaskill

Heart Attacks – Prevent and Survive
Dr Tom Smith

Helping Children Cope with Attention Deficit Disorder
Dr Patricia Gilbert

Helping Children Cope with Bullying
Sarah Lawson

Helping Children Cope with Change and Loss
Rosemary Wells

Helping Children Cope with Divorce
Rosemary Wells

Helping Children Cope with Grief
Rosemary Wells

Helping Children Cope with Stammering
Jackie Turnbull and Trudy Stewart

Helping Children Get the Most from School
Sarah Lawson

How to Accept Yourself
Dr Windy Dryden

How to Be Your Own Best Friend
Dr Paul Hauck

How to Cope with Anaemia
Dr Joan Gomez

How to Cope with Bulimia
Dr Joan Gomez

How to Cope with Stress
Dr Peter Tyrer

How to Enjoy Your Retirement
Vicky Maud

How to Improve Your Confidence
Dr Kenneth Hambly

How to Keep Your Cholesterol in Check
Dr Robert Povey

How to Lose Weight Without Dieting
Mark Barker

How to Make Yourself Miserable
Dr Windy Dryden

How to Pass Your Driving Test
Donald Ridland

How to Stand up for Yourself
Dr Paul Hauck

How to Stick to a Diet
Deborah Steinberg and Dr Windy Dryden

How to Stop Worrying
Dr Frank Tallis

The How to Study Book
Alan Brown

How to Succeed as a Single Parent
Carole Baldock

How to Untangle Your Emotional Knots
Dr Windy Dryden and Jack Gordon

Hysterectomy
Suzie Hayman

Overcoming Common Problems Series

Overcoming Common Problems

Cataract:

What You Need to Know

Mark Watts

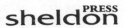
sheldon PRESS

First published in Great Britain in 2005

Sheldon Press
36 Causton Street
London SW1P 4ST

Copyright © Mark Watts 2005

The author and publisher have made every effort to ensure that the external
website and email addresses included in this book are correct and up to date at
the time of going to press. The author and publisher are not responsible for the
content, quality or continuing accessibility of the sites.

With the exception of certain case studies, the author has used 'he', 'him' and
'his' throughout. This has been done to avoid the repeated use of 'he or she'
phrases or the ungrammatical use of 'they', 'them', 'their' or 'themselves' as
singular pronouns or determiners, and is not intended to cause offence. In each
case the author intends to be non-gender-specific.

British Library Cataloguing-in-Publication Data

A catalogue record for this book is available from the British Library

ISBN 0–85969–940–4

1 3 5 7 9 10 8 6 4 2

Typeset by Deltatype Limited, Birkenhead, Merseyside
Printed in Great Britain by Ashford Colour Press

Contents

Dedication

I have never had a cataract operation. I am able to write about the experience and sensations of undergoing cataract surgery only through what the many patients I have operated on have told me. This book is dedicated to those patients.

Introduction

A single generation ago, cataract was a diagnosis feared by many, as they recalled the experiences of their friends and relatives who had suffered from either the condition or its treatment. In recent years, it has become almost something to celebrate, as people realize they have a treatable cause for their visual problems, and the expectation of a rapid and painless restoration of their sight.

Surgery used to be performed under general anaesthetic, and was followed by several weeks of hospitalization. The stay was not an easy or relaxing one, and it was necessary to observe strict bed rest, with the head immobilized with sandbags to prevent disruption of the large and sometimes painful wound. A special liquid diet was prescribed to avoid any excessive chewing action that might disturb the eye, and to loosen the bowels sufficiently to prevent any straining by the convalescent. Vision was only restored to any degree some months later, when bottle-bottomed spectacles could be ordered. Though these sometimes offered an improvement over the vision before the operation, they led to gross distortions, and the survival of eyesight at all after surgery was by no means certain. The outcome from treatment of cataract had changed very little since the earliest attempts by the Babylonians over two thousand years ago.

And then it all changed. In the 1980s, replacement of the cloudy lens or cataract by a lens implant became routine, and about a decade later the technique of removing cataract through a very small incision was developed. The combination of these two innovations transformed surgery into a routine, safe, almost painless experience. Nowadays it is usually performed as a day-case or outpatient procedure, with much improved results and a more rapid recovery. The operation can be undertaken using no anaesthetic other than drops, in a variety of settings, which include mobile units housed in lorries and dedicated cataract units, either within a hospital or standing alone. Indeed, the problem today is often not patients' fears of surgery, but their sometimes unrealistic expectations of it!

However, alongside these dramatic improvements in the management of cataract have arisen demands on patients and their relatives to make decisions. The first is whether to have surgery at all. In the past, this decision was usually not a difficult one, since operations were offered only to those with such severely impaired vision that any improvement was likely to be gratefully received. Since the cloudy lens or cataract was not replaced with an implant, there was no question of discussing the desired post-operative focus, which was largely in the hands of fate. Increased under-standing of the optics of the eye, and advances in ultrasound and other scanning equipment to measure it, now allow accurate prediction, and control, of the point of focus after surgery. Selection of a lens implant of appropriate power can modify the focus to suit the individual.

Surgery is available now to patients with often only minimal visual impairment, who face difficult decisions when weighing the potential benefits of intervention against the small, but ever present, risks. Different types of lens implants and approaches to surgery are available, as well as a range of options for both local and general anaesthesia. Other influences, such as previous laser treatment to obviate the need for glasses, which were simply not available until quite recently, can also affect the outcome, and need to be given consideration.

Although more information is available to patients now than ever before, whether this be through the media, the internet, or doctors and opticians (now known as optometrists and referred to as such throughout this book), it can still be confusing, and is not always impartial. In an age of increasing choice, even the decision as to where to go for help can be difficult. The traditional pathway of discussion with the family GP, and onward referral to the specialist of his choice, is no longer the only route. Many optometrists have direct access to hospital services, or indeed other health providers. It is not uncommon to find advertisements in newspapers and magazines for cataract surgery, allowing patients to refer themselves directly. Within the NHS in the United Kingdom, patients are increasingly being offered the option of earlier treatment at a unit they may not be familiar with, rather than remaining on the waiting list of the surgeon to whom they were initially referred. Not surprisingly, this combination of choice and information overload can be sufficient to confuse many.

The purpose of this book is to explain, in simple terms, what cataract is and the various treatment options available. The intention is to provide the reader with sufficient information to make the necessary decisions in an informed manner, and allow him or her to understand what is happening throughout the process from initial diagnosis to completion of treatment. As well as discussing routine surgery, we shall consider other options for treatment, and also study the potential risks and complications of having an operation to correct cataract, and what these mean in practical terms. The book is intended to inform not only patients with cataract, but also their families, friends and carers. We all need support when important events occur in our lives, and I hope that this book will provide it.

My experience as a surgeon has been that the more people understand their condition and its treatment, the less intimidating they find the procedure, but certain readers may wish to be selective in the detail that they read, and decide to omit, for example, studying the technical details of the operation. I know that others are fascinated by what is going on, and have many a time given a running commentary to patients undergoing surgery.

The prevailing spirit throughout this book is one of optimism. Cataract is no longer a diagnosis to be feared. It is a condition that is very amenable to treatment, if necessary, but equally it is not a diagnosis that necessarily leads to surgery. Whether an operation is necessary or not, I hope that the information contained here will provide reassurance to those experiencing cataract, and to their families and friends.

1

What is cataract?

Cataract is cloudiness of the natural lens of the eye, which is responsible for forming clear, sharply focused images on the retina. The lens normally sits in a bag, in the front one-third of the eye, as seen in Figure 1, and by altering the path of light rays passing through the clear window at the front of the eye called the cornea, brings them into focus on the retina, which in turn converts the images into signals to send to the brain. Any imperfection in the lens will obviously lead to some blurring or distortion of the image formed. If the lens has only minor imperfections, then the effects on the vision may be slight, but more marked change may cause significant loss of vision.

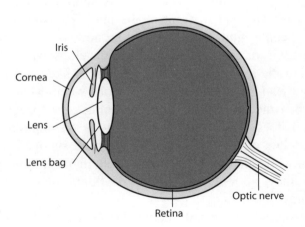

Figure 1

What are the symptoms of cataract?

The symptoms of cataract are surprisingly variable, and depend upon the nature of the change in the lens. They are often very gradual in onset, which explains why many patients develop quite advanced changes before they even recognize there is a problem.

The simple blurring of an image caused by the gradual onset of haziness in the lens may be the predominant symptom, but is often only noticed in certain lighting conditions. If the other eye is normal, however (and cataract often affects one eye more than the other, or only one eye), then the slow reduction in clarity may go completely unnoticed, until the good eye is covered over, for whatever reason, and the weakness of the eye with the cataract is noticed. Also, colours are often affected by the lens cloudiness, since it usually takes the form of a yellowish-brown discolouration and there is a consequent drab appearance of bright colours, or indeed almost complete loss of colour perception. The effect is similar to that of placing a brown filter in front of the lens of a camera.

Other people find that blurring is not so much the problem as is dazzle and glare. This develops when the structure of the lens develops changes almost like cracks in broken glass. This is usually most obvious when driving at night, when the headlights from oncoming cars appear as dazzling haloes. This is often the very first symptom of cataract, while others first notice dazzle from sunlight, and find that while they can see quite well in the home, as soon as they go out into bright daylight, their vision deteriorates.

Our modern environment imposes heavy demands on our eyes, and sometimes it is attempts to view teletext, to follow swiftly travelling golf balls at a distance, or read poor-quality newsprint that draw attention to the diagnosis. Other less common symptoms include the sensation of eye strain, headache and double vision.

It is not always the sufferer who is the one to notice cataract, however, and many people have their cataract diagnosed by their optometrists at a routine eye test. Especially when the other eye is good, and the reduced vision in the affected eye has not been noted, this may come as something of a surprise to the unsuspecting patient. The changes, which develop in the lens, can also lead to a change in its power, so that the strength of glasses needed keeps changing. Most commonly, cataract makes the eye more short-sighted – or, in other words, in focus at a point nearer than it was. Initially this might even appear to be of benefit, as some people find that they no longer need glasses to read. However, as the cataract progresses, the increased blurring makes the vision deteriorate. Optometrists are extremely good at diagnosing cataract and, if they see it and feel that treatment may be necessary, will arrange onward referral.

What causes cataract?

The most common cause of cataract is the natural degeneration of the structure of the lens that occurs with age. Exposure over the years to sunlight, and in particular the ultra-violet component of it, leads to changes in the amino acids that make up the lens proteins, and the development of bonds between them and other products that make up the lens. The effect is a gradual loss in clarity of the initially crystal-clear lens. Not surprisingly, given the role of ultra-violet light, cataract is more common in people living in areas with a lot of sunlight, such as India and Australia. Quite what the effect of the reduction in the ozone layer will be in the future remains uncertain.

In some families there is a genetic tendency towards cataract, and it is not uncommon to find a history of relatively early onset of cataract through the generations – perhaps at the age of 40 or 50. Cataract beyond the age of 60 is so common, though, that it is difficult to know whether it has developed through any genetic cause, or simply through natural ageing. Indeed, many patients who think that they have a family history of cataract really just have a family history of sufficiently good health that they live long enough to develop cataract! The condition increases in frequency with age. Studies show that 30 per cent of people over 65 have some cataract that is significantly impairing their vision. Over the age of 75 it is even more common, and in the age group 75 to 79, up to 42 per cent of people are affected.

At the other end of the age spectrum, it is possible to be born with cataract or develop it soon after birth, although this is rare. This very early-onset cataract may indicate either an hereditary lack of certain enzymes within the body, or possibly that an infection affected the unborn foetus. Certainly any very early cataract such as this should prompt investigations for a cause.

There are a number of diseases associated with cataract, the most common of which is diabetes. This is a disorder of sugar metabolism, which can occur at any age, and though most cases of cataract are nothing to do with diabetes, a simple urine test can usually make the diagnosis and is routinely undertaken in any younger patients who develop cataract.

Other diseases too specifically affect the eye and are associated with cataract. These include conditions such as uveitis, which is a recurrent inflammation within the eye, and certain types of glaucoma. Though relatively rare, these conditions may not only lead to cataract, but also present quite difficult surgical cases should treatment become necessary.

Many drugs can also precipitate or hasten the onset of cataract. In particular, steroids, which are used in the treatment of many diseases, often cause some opacity of the lens, and indeed may result in a cataract of fairly rapid onset. The degree of cataract caused is related to the dose, and people taking only small or infrequent steroids are not particularly at risk. Those requiring long-term steroids to control, for example, rheumatoid arthritis or long-standing chest diseases are much more likely to develop some visual disturbance. Steroid inhalers can lead to sufficient absorption of the drug to affect the lens, but it is more commonly steroids taken as tablets that cause cataract.

Other causes of cataract include exposure to radiation of different types. Thankfully, this is relatively uncommon, but sometimes necessary treatment for tumours around the eye may lead to cataract some years later, even when measures to protect the lens were undertaken at the time of treatment. The onset of cataract through exposure to extreme heat, as used to be seen in glass blowers and foundry workers, is now an uncommon problem.

In addition, injuries to the eye, either through accidents at work, violence, or even sometimes surgery to other parts of the eye, can all lead to cataract. In the case of an injury severe enough to pierce the coating of the eyeball, such as an assault with broken glass, cataract may develop almost immediately, and within 24 hours of the injury the lens may become completely opaque. Because of associated damage to other parts of the eye, treatment may be complicated in these cases. Therefore it is sensible to wear eye protection when undertaking tasks that could lead to eye injury, particularly when hammering or chiselling brick, stone or metal, to prevent such serious events.

Diagnosing cataract

There is a variety of ways in which cataract may be diagnosed. Although some patients may make their own diagnosis, more commonly it is the optometrist, doctor or eye specialist who will note the lens cloudiness, either at a routine examination, or if attention has been sought through the symptoms we described above. One of the advantages of eye examination is that the structures within it can normally be viewed directly. While doctors may wonder and speculate on the cause of a pain in your tummy, the reason for the actual problem is directly visible in the case of cataract. What lies behind the lens may be more difficult to assess, though, since the view into the eye is compromised for the examiner (just as the view out is for the patient), and we shall consider this in more detail later in the book.

Most often these days, cataract is diagnosed by an optometrist, and it is indeed one of the reasons why it is wise to have regular eye examinations. Once the optometrist has taken a history of the visual difficulties, the eye examination will begin with an assessment of the level of distance and reading vision. The most familiar assessment of distance vision is the chart of letters, decreasing in size from top to bottom, that we are all familiar with. This is termed a *Snellen* chart. Though seemingly a random collection of letters, it is in fact a very precisely constructed tool, which measures the fine definition that the eye can make out. Each letter is not only of an exact size, but is also made up from components of a precise size. It is the ability of the eye to see these components that allows the letter to be recognized. For example, in order to distinguish the letter 'E' from the letter 'F', the eye must be able to see the small horizontal component '_' at the base of the 'E'. This is itself of a precise length and thickness.

Depending on which line of the chart a patient is able to

see, the vision is denoted by two numbers, such as 6/12. This means that the patient can see at 6 metres (or 20 feet in imperial measurements) what he should be able to see at 12 metres. A patient with perfect vision can see 6/6 or, in other words, he can see at 6 metres what he should be able to see at 6 metres. In a non-metric scale this is 20/20, and many people still talk about 20/20 vision to mean perfect vision. In fact, many people have even better vision than this, for example 6/5 or even 6/4, especially when using both eyes together. It is not hard to work out that the letters on the line 6/12 are twice as big as those on the line 6/6.

Reading vision is assessed simply by measuring what size of print it is possible to read, with reading glasses on in good lighting, and again the size of the letters is standardized. Various notations are used, but they can all be compared with one another if necessary.

Although this measure of vision is very useful to specialists in assessing how much a patient's vision is reduced, it does not give the whole picture. We have seen earlier that some people may only be aware of their visual difficulties under certain lighting conditions. There are instruments available to measure the vision under different degrees of background lighting, but although they are useful research tools, they rarely influence the decision as to whether to operate.

Once an accurate assessment of the vision has been made, it is important to ensure that glasses worn are of the correct strength, or indeed, if glasses are not worn, to what degree they may help. Quite often an optometrist may make this assessment, and find that although the glasses may need some very slight change in power, it is cataract that is limiting the vision. He may feel that it would not be worth the time and expense to make new glasses until a decision has been made about whether cataract surgery will be undertaken, after consultation with an eye specialist. Since glasses usually need changing after eye surgery, it is clearly not sensible to make up a new pair if surgery is likely and imminent, until this has been completed.

Often a cataract can easily be seen by direct examination of the eye simply with a light, but it is usual to look more closely using a type of microscope called a slit-lamp. This device projects a slit of light to illuminate the eye, which the examiner views through a set of eyepieces similar to binoculars. The patient simply places his chin on a rest. To enhance the view of the lens and eye behind, he may instil some eye drops, which widen the pupil approximately fifteen minutes later, when he can repeat the examination. These wear off after a few hours, but leave the vision rather blurred while this is happening. For this reason, it is not advisable to drive until the effect has completely worn off, and you would always be advised of the impending blur before the eye drops were given.

Diagnosis of cataract, then, is usually fairly straightforward. What such a diagnosis means is quite variable, though, and we shall now consider the implications in different situations, and how it should be managed.

2

So do I need an operation?

Once the diagnosis of cataract has been made, the question of what to do next arises. Not all cataract requires surgery, and deciding how to proceed involves weighing up the risks and benefits, and considering what is likely to happen without any treatment, as well as the likely outcome from having surgery. Although treatment usually does involve an operation, some benefit can be achieved in certain cases from glasses or even eye drops. In this chapter we will consider the factors involved in making the decision as to how to manage cataract.

Some common myths

It is helpful first to dispel a number of misunderstandings, which have grown up over the years into the folklore of cataract treatment.

The most common of these is that there is a critical 'time window' during which surgery must be undertaken, and that it is necessary to allow a cataract to become 'ripe' before surgery is safe. This is absolutely not the case with modern surgery, but the myth originates from the days when the operation involved squeezing out the lens intact from the eye, through a relatively large incision. If the cataract was at an early stage, and the lens therefore still soft, the surgery could be more hazardous. In addition, the results of surgery were often so poor that it could not be recommended until the vision was so reduced that the final result would be an improvement on the relatively unsatisfactory results then achieved! Thankfully, this situation has now changed. Good results can be expected from surgery, and the lens is removed through a small incision by turning it into a fluid. It is actually easier, and somewhat safer, to undertake surgery before the lens has become very thick and opaque, although surgery is now possible at all stages of cataract development. The indication for an operation is when the cataract is causing a problem, and when the likely benefits outweigh the small risks involved.

Another common misapprehension is that the benefit from surgery will only last for a certain time. Many people believe that after, say, ten years, the lens implant, which is inserted in place of the natural lens, which is removed, will wear out. Again, this is not true, and presumably derives from the fact that certain implants, such as those used in hip surgery, do have a limited life. Lens implants remain functional for the rest of the patient's life, and indeed beyond. Morbid thought as it may be, the lens implants that are inserted nowadays will still be in perfect condition when our descendants dig up our bones in centuries to come. One wonders what they will make of them!

The misconceptions as to how surgery is actually undertaken are too numerous and gruesome to describe. In truth, modern cataract surgery is probably the most elegant operation currently undertaken, and is completely bloodless. Those who have seen it performed usually marvel at the delicacy and finesse involved, and it is far removed from the imaginative but inaccurate descriptions often proffered by helpful friends, neighbours or relatives. Details of the surgery are described later in this book.

Having dispelled some myths, let us return to the considerations we need to make in deciding the best way forward in management of cataract.

How much is the cataract affecting my vision?

This question is obviously key in deciding what best to do about cataract, since we have already seen that a minor change in the lens, which could quite accurately be described as cataract, may have no effect on the vision, and therefore require no treatment. At the opposite extreme, a dense cataract causing severe loss of vision is probably best treated surgically, assuming the rest of the eye appears healthy after examination. Most cataracts are somewhere between these two extremes, and the first consideration in deciding treatment is the degree to which vision is affected.

Symptoms, which were considered in the previous chapter, are as important a part of this assessment as are accurate measurements of visual function undertaken by an optometrist or eye specialist. Many people with early cataract and good vision on a test chart may still be troubled sufficiently by glare to wish to proceed with surgery, while others, who perhaps are happy to give up driving at night, may not wish to have treatment.

It is helpful, however, to have some repeatable measure of vision function, not only to help in the decision as to whether to have surgery, but also to measure its success. In Chapter 1 we saw how vision can be assessed and recorded. Increasingly, optometrists and eye specialists rely not only on the results from these sorts of tests, but also on patients' symptoms, and so systems of scoring symptoms in a repeatable manner have been devised. These ask specific, standardized questions about what the visual difficulties are. Though not widespread yet, they are in increasing use, and a valuable aid to assessment.

Cataract often occurs in elderly people, and so, unfortunately, do other eye diseases. Therefore in order to work out how much cataract is affecting the vision, it is necessary to assess also the effect of other diseases, and indeed the effect of the natural ageing process. It is normal, for instance, for the retina, and in particular the central part of it termed the macula, to become less sensitive with age, and less able to discern fine detail. The retina is responsible for translating focused images into electrical signals to send to the brain, and if the retina becomes less sensitive, then so in turn will the signals be less clear. We shall consider the effects of other conditions on vision in the next chapter.

Is it the cataract alone that is affecting my vision?

It is a common assumption that cataract, if present, is the sole cause of vision problems, and therefore that its treatment will fully resolve the matter. Often this is indeed the case, but many people with cataract have other factors influencing their vision. Therefore part of the assessment of a patient for surgery involves identifying any other conditions, which might either limit the effectiveness of surgery, or indeed make it not worthwhile at all. Conditions such as glaucoma, diabetic eye disease and macular degeneration may all lead to less than perfect outcomes from surgery, even though there may still be significant improvement in the vision. If we think of the eye as a camera, with a lens and a film, there will obviously be only limited improvement in the quality of the pictures if a new lens is used to replace an old one, if the *film* (the equivalent of which in the eye is the retina) is poor.

Other factors, which are simpler to correct, may also be involved. The most obvious one of these is the spectacle correction that is being worn, or indeed not worn. Cataract can change the power of the lens, and therefore the strength of glasses needed. Sometimes this is the only effect it has on the eye, and the only treatment needed is a change in glasses. Even more simply, I have on occasion 'cured' patients by cleaning their glasses, or fixing the lens back in the spectacle frame!

What will happen if I don't have surgery?

Many people request operations for cataract more in fear of what might happen if they do nothing, than as a solution to a current problem. It is a mistake to undergo an operation in anticipation of a situation that may never arise, since we know that many cataracts do not progress at all – or progress so slowly that they never become a problem. It may, of course, be difficult for the patient, or indeed the specialist, to predict the likely speed of deterioration of vision, but there are certain types of cataract that are likely to progress more rapidly than others. It is certainly worth asking your specialist if he can give any idea of how quickly the cataract might change. It is, however, a reasonable assumption that any cataract, once formed, will not disappear of its own accord, and that any change in vision is likely to be for the worse. In addition, as a cataract progresses, it often changes the power of the eye, such that more frequent changes in glasses may be necessary. Most patients find they need their glasses changing less frequently once cataract has been dealt with, than they did while it was still progressing.

We have seen that with modern surgery it is neither necessary to delay operation until a certain cloudiness has developed, nor to rush into it before the cataract reaches any critical point. Surgery can be undertaken at any stage of cataract development, and it is even possible to remove a normal lens that does not have cataract, in exceptional circumstances (reasons for doing this will be given later). It is therefore perfectly reasonable, if you are undecided, to just wait and see what happens without treatment. If your vision continues to fail, the decision may become much easier, while if it is maintained at the same level, many people will decide to avoid surgery as long as they are managing well. Although the risks involved in surgery remain broadly unchanged as a cataract progresses (unless it progresses to total blackout of vision), the relative benefits increase as the vision fails. For example, somebody who has a very advanced cataract that stops them driving, reading or maintaining their independence, is likely to notice recovery to 6/6 vision more than somebody who already has 6/6 vision, but who has early cataract interfering with their golf on a sunny day! Although the risks may be the same for the two operations, the first patient has more to gain (and less to lose) than the second. It is this weighing of the risks and benefits that is the final determinant of whether to have an operation. Your specialist, optometrist, friends and neighbours can all advise and help, but it is the patient who ultimately has to make the final decision.

The alternatives to surgery

So what are the alternatives to an operation, and under which circumstances are they advisable?

The most obvious alternative is to do nothing. This may sound like the proverbial ostrich sticking its head in the sand and hoping the problem will go away, but is a perfectly reasonable approach if either the cataract is genuinely causing no problem, or if the other options are really not acceptable. Very few patients are too infirm or too old to undergo surgery, however. I have operated on many patients still attached to their oxygen cylinders that they need to use constantly to keep them breathing, and also on a 103-year-old! So although factors of age or other illness should not therefore rule out surgery, 'leaving well alone' is certainly an option that some people will choose.

'Could I not just have stronger glasses?' is a question

asked frequently by patients with cataract, the short answer to which is 'No'. Thinking of the camera analogy again, it is easy to understand that just putting a stronger lens in front of a lens that has become scratched or cloudy will not solve the problem. If the cataract is fairly early, though, and so far has only had the effect of changing the power of the lens, then stronger, or indeed weaker, glasses may help. Glasses as an alternative to surgery is rarely a good option, but as a compromise may suit some people.

Under rare circumstances, in which the cataract affects only a small, central portion of the lens, it may be possible to improve the vision by instilling drops that widen the pupil, and allow vision 'around' the cloudy part of the lens. Unfortunately, the drops used to widen the pupil also paralyse the focusing muscles within the eye, need to be used continuously, and give only a marginal improvement.

There are intermittent reports in the media of drops to dissolve cataract. The concept is attractive, even to a surgeon who earns his living by operating on them! So far, the usefulness of such drops in the management of cataract remains uncertain, and further trials will be needed if they are to play a significant part in treatment.

It will already be apparent that different plans for management are appropriate for different people. Quite apart from the differences in the nature of the cataract and other variables within the eye, we are all different in character, and what we are troubled by, or indeed what risks we are prepared to take. Patients often ask if they are 'doing the right thing' in making the decision either to have surgery or not, and worry that they might not be conforming to some imaginary norm of behaviour. What is right for one person may not be right for another. Let us consider some case histories that illustrate this.

Peter

Peter is 76 and had become aware of some slight blurring of his vision over the last few months. Most of the time he was not greatly troubled by this, but found his distance vision in dim light was somewhat reduced. His near vision remained good, and he had found that recently, as long as he had good lighting, he could even see quite well without wearing his reading glasses, which he had needed for about thirty years. He attended his routine annual visit to his optometrist, and was somewhat surprised to be told that he had early cataract. His optometrist informed him that, on testing, his vision was 6/9, still well within the standard for driving.

After discussion with his optometrist, Peter felt that he was not sufficiently troubled by the modest reduction in vision to wish onward referral for surgery, and decided to leave well alone. With a new pair of glasses his distance vision was improved. His optometrist kept a watch on him, and saw him six months later, and his vision and glasses remained unchanged. Two years later he had still suffered no deterioration, and remains under annual review by his optometrist.

Peter's case illustrates a number of common features of cataract. The first is that he was relatively little troubled by it, and could still manage to drive safely and undertake his daily activities without a problem. His ability to read without his reading glasses suggests that the cataract was making the eye a little bit short-sighted – or, in other words, bringing his point of focus nearer. Most people find that in middle age and beyond, they have to hold things further away to bring them into focus. The change in focus caused by the cataract was in this case actually beneficial, at least for reading. Peter could quite reasonably have elected to have an operation, and he would probably have found an improvement in the brightness of colours, and some increased sharpness. His decision was to leave things. Although in another few years' time he may find that the cataract has progressed, he still has the option to have surgery then.

Barbara

Barbara is 72 and lives alone. She had been aware of a gradually increasing difficulty with both distance and reading vision over a period of approximately eighteen months, but more particularly over the last three months. She went to see her optometrist expecting to be given stronger glasses, but she informed her that her vision was reduced as a result of cataract in both eyes, more marked on the right.

Barbara realized that if her vision deteriorated further she would not be able to remain independent, and decided to go forward to surgery. After discussion with her surgeon, she decided to have an operation on the right eye first, which was performed under local anaesthesia. Her vision improved from 6/60 (the top line of the vision chart) to 6/6 ('normal' vision), following which she was so delighted that she asked for surgery to the left eye. Although the sharpness of vision took several weeks to fully recover and she needed a change to her glasses, she became aware of improvement within 24 hours of the surgery. She couldn't believe how colours had become so bright, and decided to redecorate her front room, which wasn't the colour she had thought it was!

What a happy ending! This case history is quite typical of patients who have surgery, although obviously not every operation can be guaranteed to restore 6/6 vision. There was little difficulty for Barbara in deciding to have an operation. Her vision was poor, and her independence threatened. She

17

felt she had 'nothing to lose'. In fact, she did have something to lose: she could have lost the small amount of vision she had in that right eye, if she had been unlucky enough to suffer an extremely rare, serious complication, and we shall discuss such events later in the book. She knew, however, that left untreated the eye was likely to continue to deteriorate, and the three months before surgery had seen a significant decline in her vision. In addition, if the worst happened, and she did have a problem with her right eye, she knew that she still had some useful vision in the left, with which she might manage – even if not with the same degree of independence she had been used to. Barbara had weighed up the very small risks of a problem as a result of surgery, and the consequences of it, against the much more likely outcome of dramatically improved vision, and decided to have an operation. She was delighted that she had made the right decision.

Christine

Christine first noted problems with her vision at the age of 53. Although she had been wearing reading glasses for seven years, she began to notice difficulty driving at night, and was finding the dazzle from oncoming headlights increasingly difficult to cope with. She worked as a busy sales executive, and feared that she might have problems coping with this if the vision deteriorated any further. Her father had suffered cataract at a relatively early age, but had not had a good result from surgery, and she was very nervous about any intervention. Christine enjoyed tennis, but was finding that her game had deteriorated recently, which she felt was because of some difficulty in seeing the ball in bright sunlight.

Her optometrist identified cataract in her right eye, just in the centre of the back surface of the lens. Her vision on the eye chart was still good at 6/6. After a long discussion with her surgeon, she finally decided to have surgery to the right eye. After the operation, her vision was still 6/6, but she no longer noticed the glare at night, and her tennis improved. She still needed reading glasses, but overall she felt that her level of vision was much better.

This was not an easy decision for Christine, particularly in view of her father's poor outcome from surgery many years previously, but she had a good result. Her case illustrates clearly that improving the line on the chart that can be read is not the only measure of success or otherwise of the operation. Christine was still only reading the same line (albeit the bottom but one on the chart), after the operation as she was before, but her symptoms of glare and dazzle were improved. Compared with Peter, she had better vision even before surgery than he did, as assessed by the vision chart, but was more troubled by her symptoms. She chose to have surgery, while he was happy not to. Whereas Peter could do all he wanted to with his level of vision, Christine was having difficulty both holding down her job and enjoying her tennis. Peter and Christine both made the correct decision for them, and this is what is really important.

Decisions can be difficult, and some people find decision-making more difficult than others. Perhaps Christine was used to taking difficult decisions in her high-pressure job, but even the toughest decision-makers who are used to such challenges sometimes have difficulty in deciding what is right for them. Indeed, such personalities are often the ones who are least certain about what to do when it comes to their own decisions!

Do not be worried by this. By all means, consult the people whose opinions you respect, whether they be professionals or friends and family, but remember that ultimately *you* are the one who has to either live with the cataract, or undergo the operation.

3

Assessment before the operation

Optometrists are very skilled at diagnosing and assessing cataract, but before the final decision to undertake surgery is made, it is usual for further tests to be undertaken at the unit where the surgery will be performed. Traditionally this has been a hospital, although in recent years there has been an increase in the variety and location of cataract units. Whatever the nature of the location, certain pre-operative assessments need to be undertaken.

Broadly speaking, these can be divided into two parts: a further medical assessment of the eye and the patient, and specific measurements of the eye which are necessary to choose the power of the lens implant that will be inserted at the time of surgery.

Medical assessment

Increasingly, optometrists and eye specialists work together to share information, and much of what used to be carried out in the hospital has now already been done by the optometrist by the time of referral. However, there are specific aspects of the medical history and examination that a surgeon will wish to know before surgery.

Although the optometrist or referring doctor will have provided some details of the previous history, an eye assessment will usually begin with an enquiry into the nature of the visual problem, and any relevant past eye history. In particular, any previous eye diseases are relevant. Some people have always had some weakness of one or other eye since birth, and it is useful to know this in order to assess if surgery is likely to aid vision, or whether the 'lazy' eye has only limited potential for improvement. Other specific previous eye diseases such as glaucoma, uveitis or repeated infections may also be important. Of increasing relevance is whether there has been any previous laser surgery to the eye to treat long- or short-sight. This is not always apparent on examination, and you should inform the surgeon if you have had such surgery, since account needs to be taken of this in calculating the power of the lens implant.

A surgeon will also be interested in your general health. This is because some diseases, most obviously diabetes, will affect the eye, but also it is important to know about any general health factors that may influence how the surgery is undertaken. Patients with a bad tremor, for example, may not be able to keep sufficiently still for surgery to be performed under local anaesthetic.

Any medications that you are taking are both relevant and important, and in particular drugs used to thin the blood, such as warfarin. Again, these may influence how the surgery is done, and what form of anaesthesia to use.

The examination undertaken at the cataract unit will probably repeat some of the assessments that have already been made by the referring optometrist or doctor. However, it is normal to measure the vision again, particularly if there has been any delay between initial referral and the assessment.

Following this, the eyes are examined, with attention being paid not only to the eye itself, but to the eyelids also. If the lids are poorly positioned, infected or inflamed, it may be necessary to deal with this first, in order to minimize any chances of infection after surgery.

An examination of the eye using the slit-lamp is then performed as described earlier. The surgeon will be concentrating particularly on identifying any factors that may either make the surgery more difficult or dangerous, or may be likely to influence the final result. Certain conditions of the cornea, for example, make it more likely that vision might become hazy after surgery. This will influence the approach to surgery, or in extreme cases even make it inadvisable altogether. The pressure of the eye is checked to screen for glaucoma, and the pupils are examined. If a pupil will not open wide following insertion of drops, then the surgery is considerably more complex and hazardous. Again, these are factors that the surgeon will want to know about before the operation.

Although, as we mentioned earlier, a thick cataract will prevent as good a view into the eye as might be ideal, it is usual to be able to make some assessment of the back of the eye. In doing so it is possible to identify any conditions that may limit the success of surgery. The most common of these is macular degeneration, which can range enormously in severity. This is not in itself a reason not to undertake surgery, but may limit the improvement to be expected.

It is important also, of course, to make an assessment of the lens itself, since this is the part of the eye that is to be operated upon. Sometimes the degree of cloudiness of the lens does not match the reduction in vision experienced by the patient, and this may prompt further examination or investigation to assess if there is any other disease limiting the vision.

If the lens is so opaque as to prevent any view into the eye, it may be helpful to perform an ultrasound test. This simply involves placing a sensor (which is rather like a thick pencil) on the eye, which is covered in a sort of jelly, to image the inside of it just as an obstetrician would look at an unborn baby in a pregnant woman. It is painless. Although it gives some idea of the structure within the eye, and would for example identify a retinal detachment, it does not give an assessment of how well the eye will function.

At the conclusion of these examinations it is possible to get an idea of what particular problems, if any, might be anticipated during surgery, and plan any appropriate action to avoid them. In addition, some idea of the likely outcome has been gained, and if there is any reason why this might be poor – such as other disease having been detected – this can be discussed. It is often helpful at this stage to discuss also the type of anaesthetic that will be used, and we shall consider this in some detail in the next chapter.

The second stage of the assessment before surgery is the measurement of the eyes for the specific purpose of selecting the lens implant power. These measurements are termed *biometry*.

Biometry

In the early years of lens implantation after cataract extraction, selection of lens implant power was a very imprecise process. Surgeons knew that an individual who was short-sighted before surgery generally needed a less powerful lens implant than somebody who was long-sighted, but beyond this there was an element of guesswork and good fortune. Over the years, however, techniques have been developed that predict much more accurately what power of lens implant will lead to a particular point of focus in any specific eye.

The two principal determinants of the lens power needed are the length of the eyeball, from the front of the cornea to the retina, and the curvature of the cornea. It is these measurements that are made during biometry. When these measurements are fed into a complex mathematical formula (thankfully now calculated by computers!), a prediction of the appropriate lens power can be made. Unfortunately, people are not as uniform as mathematical models, and there can still be deviations from the predictions. However, increasingly accurate formulae, and audit of the results achieved, have made the process reasonably accurate now. It is still not possible to choose the point of focus to within a few centimetres, but it is usually possible to select a lens power sufficiently accurately to choose that the focus be for distance, for example, or near if this is preferable.

There are a number of ways in which to assess the corneal curvature and the length of the eye. Although the precise details vary between different machines, most commonly the curvature of the cornea is assessed by viewing the reflected images of light projected on to the front of the eye. This does not involve contact with the eye, and is therefore painless. Although the technique is extremely accurate, it may be difficult to get clear readings if the cornea is scarred, and can give misleading readings if there has been previous refractive laser surgery. (Refractive laser surgery is laser to treat long- or short-sight, as opposed to laser for treatment of, for example, diabetes or macular disease.)

The length of the eye is usually measured using ultrasound. In this technique a small probe, about the size of a short pencil, is placed on the surface of the cornea, and emits ultrasound waves. The time is measured for the wave to reach into the eye, and be reflected back to the probe by the retina. Knowing the speed that the wave travels within the eye, it is possible to calculate the distance from the front of the cornea to the retina. Before the examination, anaesthetic drops are placed in the eye, so that it is painless. A variant of the technique is to create a small water bath around the eye, and place the probe in this. This can be more accurate in some cases, but is somewhat messier!

Recently, instruments have been developed that take the same measurements using laser light rather than ultrasound. These have the advantage of requiring no direct physical contact with the eye, but are not suitable for all cataracts.

Biometry is a critical step in preparation for surgery, since insertion of the wrong power of implant will not provide the intended visual result. In the rare cases of biometry error, whether this be through inaccurate measurement, or through the fact that the operated eye has not conformed to the formula, it may even be necessary to remove the implant and exchange it for another, or to insert a second implant on top of the first.

Different Eye Units have varying arrangements for the measurements and assessments that need to be made before surgery. If general anaesthesia is being considered, it may be necessary to also take blood samples, a chest X-ray and an ECG reading of the heart. In addition, it is necessary to discuss what the process will involve and make plans for post-operative care. In particular, it is helpful in advance to be thinking about how to get home after the operation, whether you will be able to put the drops in yourself, and how you will manage in the immediate post-operative period. Relatives, friends and neighbours can all be of enormous help, and it is worth approaching them early to ask for any support that they might be able to give.

Another key question to think about before surgery is the type of anaesthetic to be used, and it is important that both the patient and surgeon have input into this decision. It is this topic that we shall study next.

4
Types of anaesthetic

A variety of different types of anaesthetic are available for cataract surgery. These range from simply placing anaesthetic drops in the eye, to a full general anaesthetic. Selection of the best type of anaesthetic depends upon the type of cataract and the preferences and health of the patient, as well as the choice of the surgeon. Before discussing this in more detail, let us consider the types of anaesthetic currently in use.

Categories of anaesthetic

Local anaesthetic injection

This has been the most common form of anaesthetic used for cataract surgery for some years. Although the thought of an injection around the eye seems unpleasant, it is not as disagreeable as it might sound and is an extremely effective way of rapidly achieving complete numbness of the eye, allowing painless surgery. The injection is not into the eye itself, but into the soft tissues around it.

Before the injection is given, drops are put into the eye to numb these tissues, rather as the dentist may spray the mouth with anaesthetic before an injection. The injection itself is a little uncomfortable for a few moments, but it is rare to have any severe pain, and it is short-lived. Although the vision usually goes very hazy soon afterwards, most eyes still have some perception of light, but it is not possible to see any of the operation anyway because the microscope light blinds the eye temporarily through its intense brightness. The anaesthetic not only numbs the eye, but also prevents it moving around, which is helpful to the surgeon. It usually takes a few hours to wear off, and it is common during this period to experience double vision while the muscles that move the eye are recovering.

The technique is very safe and effective, but there are certain disadvantages. Perhaps the main one is the very small risk of bleeding being caused by the needle as the injection is undertaken. The eye socket is full of blood vessels, and if one of these is pierced by the anaesthetic needle (and it is not possible for the person giving the anaesthetic to see them), then it may bleed. This can cause a sudden bulging of the eye, which requires the surgery to be postponed. Even more rarely, the bleeding may be sufficient that it is necessary to make a small cut into the eye socket to relieve the pressure. Intense pressure could damage the eye permanently. Clearly, there are enhanced risks with this technique in people taking blood-thinning agents such as warfarin, which may need to be stopped before surgery if this technique is to be used.

There are also very small risks of damaging the eyeball itself with the needle. Though this is an extremely rare complication, it can have serious implications, and is more likely in very short-sighted people.

Finally, because the vision is also frozen by the injection, it is a few hours before the eye can see. This is not a big problem in patients with two seeing eyes, since the other can be used to navigate while the eye recovers. In patients having surgery to their only seeing eye, though, this period of complete blindness for a few hours can be difficult and distressing.

In spite of these risks and side effects, the technique is tried and tested, and has been used millions of times with very few problems. Currently, it is still one of the most common forms of local anaesthetic.

Sub-tenon local anaesthetic injection

In an attempt to gain the advantages of a local anaesthetic injection, but reduce the risks of bleeding or damage to the eyeball, a technique of anaesthetic termed *sub-tenon* injection has been developed. Essentially, this is similar to the use of a local anaesthetic injection, but instead of using a needle to inject through the tissues around the eye into the eye socket, the local anaesthetic is given by means of a slightly bent and flattened, blunt, round pipe, of calibre somewhat thicker than a hypodermic needle. It is introduced through a small cut in the conjunctiva, covering the eyeball, which has previously been frozen with drops. The pipe is then used to direct the local anaesthetic under a layer of connective tissue that wraps around the eye; this is called *Tenon's capsule* – hence the name of the technique.

The advantage of this over a needle injection is that the risks of bleeding and damage to the eyeball are reduced. It completely avoids the use of a needle, but the other limitations of the technique still exist. Although it has some advantages, opinion is still somewhat divided among surgeons as to which method is preferable. Some surgeons feel that the reduction in movement of the eye is more consistent with needle anaesthesia, and others are simply more familiar with one technique over the other.

Anaesthetic drops only

It is perfectly possible to undertake cataract surgery in most people simply by putting drops into their eye, and this simplest of anaesthetics has many advantages, and is my own preferred technique. It is often termed *topical* anaesthesia. It avoids all the risks of the two types of anaesthesia discussed above, and in addition provides an almost instant recovery of some vision after surgery. The problem of double vision during recovery does not exist, and it is safe for people on blood-thinning agents such as warfarin, since no blood vessels are touched. It does not, however, provide the absolute numbness that an injection will, nor does it paralyse the muscles that move the eye. The eye is still not able to see the operation, because the intense bleaching of the eye by the microscope light prevents this. Although most patients do not experience any discomfort, it is normal for there to be some sensation of pressure at certain points in the operation. The technique is well suited to people with no vision in the other eye, or to those who are very short-sighted, in whom the risks of damaging the eyeball with a needle, or even the blunt pipe, are avoided.

The technique is not right for everybody. Patients who are extremely anxious and squeeze their eyelids hard together are usually not ideal candidates for this form of anaesthetic. Equally, some surgeons do not like using the technique, particularly if more manipulations than usual are likely to be needed for the operation. This might be the case if, for example, there is a small pupil that requires stretching to facilitate removal of the lens.

Barbara again

Barbara, whose decision to have surgery we considered earlier, had surgery using drops alone as an anaesthetic. She was keen to have a local, since she had heard favourable reports from her friends, but knew nothing of the details of different types of local. She had been on warfarin to thin her blood ever since an episode of irregular heart rhythm, and for this reason she and her specialist decided that topical anaesthetic would be best for her. She found this not to be unpleasant at all, although she was aware of a sensation of pressure at some points during the operation. In addition, she noticed coloured shapes and lights. She was surprised that even five minutes after the surgery she could already see a little out of the eye. She was collected and taken home by a friend one hour after the operation, and felt it had been 'not as bad as going to the dentist'!

This form of anaesthesia was fine for Barbara, as it is for most patients, and she benefited from the very rapid recovery achieved with drops alone. In addition, the avoidance of any form of needle meant that there was no need for her to stop her warfarin.

Local anaesthetic with sedation

Most patients feel anxious while having surgery, and this is both normal and understandable. But some patients are so anxious that they are not able to co-operate sufficiently to allow safe surgery. Under these circumstances, it may be helpful to administer some form of sedation. Although this may take the form of a tablet before the operation, more commonly these days an injection into a blood vessel in the arm is given, which has a very rapid effect in bringing about whatever level of sedation is required – from mild calming to almost being asleep. This requires careful administration and monitoring by an anaesthetist, and does lead to some drowsiness afterwards for a while. If this is to be used, it is best to starve beforehand as for a general anaesthetic.

Sedation can be used in combination with any of the forms of local anaesthetic described above. It has traditionally not been widespread as routine in the United Kingdom, although it is very popular in the United States.

General anaesthetic

Although this was once the routine technique of anaesthesia for cataract surgery, general anaesthesia is now used in a relatively small number of operations. It still has a place, however, and the drugs and techniques used are far advanced from those of even ten or fifteen years ago. Modern drugs give rapid recovery, usually allowing return home on the day of surgery, just as if local anaesthetic had been used, and the sore throats and vomiting that people feared from general anaesthesia are very rare these days.

Usually the choice of a general anaesthetic is at the patient's request, but there are circumstances under which the surgeon may prefer the technique. These are usually if he feels that the patient might not be able to keep sufficiently still, perhaps because he is not able to lie on the couch through bad arthritis, or if there is a bad, uncontrollable tremor due to Parkinson's disease. Sometimes the surgery itself might be a reason for a general anaesthetic: if it is likely to be particularly complex or hazardous, and complete immobility of the eye is required for a longer period than normal.

Many patients who think that they want to be asleep for the surgery do so because they have misunderstandings about local anaesthetic. Many of these, once they understand what actually is involved, will very happily have a local anaesthetic with a good result, but there are still some who really cannot face this prospect and choose a general anaesthetic. Some of these then worry unnecessarily that they have failed or 'chickened out'.

The reason there are various techniques of anaesthetic is that there are different personalities of patient (and indeed surgeon) and different clinical situations, both in terms of the cataract itself and the general physical health of the patient. The important thing is to consider what is best for the particular patient and their clinical situation in order to choose what is right.

It is not possible to generalize, but in my own practice I find that the patients for whom we choose a general anaesthetic are usually the younger ones (under 45), the more frail, those who find it hard to lie down comfortably, and those who have just decided that this is the only technique for them!

The risks of general anaesthesia are small, but there are

rare circumstances where, after consultation with the anaesthetist, this form of anaesthetic might be declined. Other patients may need specific investigations beforehand, such as an ECG or even ultrasound examination of the heart, depending on their previous medical history.

It is important if you are having a general anaesthetic to be starved beforehand. Although the unit will probably issue specific instructions, which you should follow, this usually means no food for at least six hours before surgery, and no fluids for at least four hours. It is not advisable to drink alcohol for 24 hours after a general anaesthetic, nor to operate any machinery, which obviously includes driving.

Christine again

Christine was very nervous about her decision to have cataract surgery. As we read earlier, her father had had complications many years previously, and although she knew that things had changed since those days, she could not get it out of her mind that something might go wrong. She had attempted to wear contact lenses in the past, but had never been comfortable with them as she found the thought of inserting and removing them quite upsetting. She was the first to admit to being a coward, and felt she could not possibly have surgery while awake. So she chose to have a general anaesthetic, but was still able to go home on the day of her surgery, which took place during the afternoon. Her husband collected her from hospital, and she rested quietly at home that evening. The following day she felt fine, and returned to work two days later.

Most people feel nervous about surgery, and this is not in itself a reason to opt for a general anaesthetic. However, Christine's anxieties, caused mainly by her father's previous history, and her very sensitive eyes which had given her trouble with contact lenses in the past, added up to make an operation under local anaesthetic unacceptable to her. She was not being a coward – she was simply choosing the best type of anaesthetic for her. She did very well, and was even back at work within two days. Although many people may feel they need a little more recovery time than this, modern general anaesthetics allow rapid return to normal activity.

To sum up, there is no 'correct' or 'best' type of anaesthetic, and individual surgeons will almost certainly have their own preferences too. However, it is important that, whatever form of anaesthesia you have, you understand what is about to happen – since knowing about it in advance is the best way to allay anxieties. Although even now some people request 'not to know anything about it – just get on and treat me!', these are rarely the most relaxed patients. Even if you feel like this, if you can attempt some understanding of what goes on, life becomes easier. If you have managed to read this far, you have already achieved this.

5

Countdown to surgery

The days or weeks before surgery offer a useful opportunity to make final arrangements to make the whole process as smooth and easy as possible. We will now consider some of the things that need to be organized before your admission. If need be, write yourself a checklist of things to do, so that you do not need to worry that you have forgotten something.

Preparations at the Eye Unit

During the few weeks before your operation, you will have had measurements of your eyes taken (biometry), and any other assessments necessary, as we have discussed earlier. Although all units have slightly different details for the precise timing of these events, you should have had a chance to ask any questions you may have about the operation, and in most cases will have been given a leaflet to explain what goes on. If you still have any questions, this is the time to ask. At some stage you will be asked to sign a consent form, to demonstrate that you understand what you are about to have done, and agree to it. Obviously you can only do this if you have the necessary information. Although this book should hopefully provide all the information that you need to know about cataract surgery, there are individual differences between units in how things are done.

Patients sometimes worry about the consent form, while others do not read it at all. Some people fear that it is a licence for the surgeon to do whatever he wants, regardless of the consequences, and that it is a disclaimer should anything go wrong. This is absolutely not the case, and the fact that specific complications may have been mentioned on it does not in any way absolve all those involved in your care from their obligations to minimize the risks of complications or deal with the consequences of them. The consent form is simply a formal acknowledgement by the patient that he is in agreement with the proposed treatment, and wishes to go ahead with it, and a formal acknowledgement by the surgeon that he has explained the procedure and its implications.

Preparations at home

There are not a lot of preparations to make at home before surgery, since the procedure is generally done as a day admission, and in this respect you can consider your cataract operation as just another day out! Admittedly, certain aspects of the day are different from a day trip, and may need some planning:

How will you get to and from the Eye Unit?

It is not safe to drive home after an eye operation, even if it has been done under local anaesthetic, and plans need to be made for transport. Ideally, somebody may be able to take you and collect you from the hospital in a car. If so, it is important that they know when you should arrive, and also at roughly what time they should be ready to pick you up. If this is not possible, then it may be necessary for you to travel by ambulance, and again these arrangements need to be made in advance. You should discuss these with the Eye Unit if there is any doubt. The same consideration should be made for follow-up arrangements. Some units like to review patients on the first day after surgery, and you may need transport for this.

Do you need any help when you arrive home?

Many patients live alone, and return to an empty home. Although this is not advisable if you are having a general anaesthetic as a day case procedure, there is no reason why a patient having surgery under local anaesthetic should not return home on the same day. However, patients who have been put to sleep for the surgery should have somebody with them on the first night following the operation.

If you will be returning to an empty home, it is worth considering how you will manage for the first night. Will you be able to prepare a meal, or could somebody bring something round for you? Should you prepare a meal in advance? Obviously the answers to these questions depend upon a number of factors. In particular, the vision in the other eye is significant. If it has good vision, then even if the operated eye is still blurred some hours after the operation, you will be likely to manage; but if the other eye is completely blind, life may be a little difficult for at least several hours. If this is the case, you should consider whether you will be able to manage alone at home for the first few hours. If you are not able, then consider if somebody might be able to help, or even whether a friend, neighbour or family member might be able to have you to stay with them for the night. Although not all units have facilities for an overnight stay, they may be able to help, or even make hotel arrangements for you.

Are there any arrangements that need to be made at home?

Most people can leave home for the day without too much planning, but if you do have dependants, they may need catering for. Some patients care for others in their home, and it may be necessary to arrange for, for example, a disabled husband to have respite care or support from somebody else for a short time. It is clearly not advisable to return home from an operation and start lifting somebody in and out of bed on the same day, and you may need to make arrangements for this. Others may need to make arrangements for their pets.

The day of surgery

On the day of surgery, make sure that you have read any instructions issued by the unit you are to attend. The guidelines below are those that I advise to my patients, but if these differ from those given by your unit, follow closely what the local unit has requested.

Clothes

Many units allow patients to wear their own clothes during surgery under local anaesthetic, rather than wear a hospital gown. If this is the case, wear something comfortable rather than glamorous. Cataract surgery involves a lot of irrigation with water, and it is possible for some to leak on to your neck during the operation. Although it is only sterile water, be prepared for this, and even consider taking a change of shirt. It is a good idea to wear clothes that can be unbuttoned at the front to attach chest monitors if these are used. For men this is usually simple, but women should consider wearing a shirt or blouse rather than a dress. If you are staying overnight, take appropriate clothing, together with basic toiletries.

Do not apply make-up on the day of surgery. Although you may feel awkward going out without it, it will only have to be removed from your lids at the time of operation, and may make the lids more difficult to clean.

Medication and eye drops

If you are on regular medication, you should continue this as normal, unless otherwise advised. This includes any eye drops you are using. In most cases, the unit will want you to continue as normal, but you may be asked to stop blood-thinning drugs such as warfarin. Diabetics who are having a general anaesthetic will need specific advice about their medication since they will need to alter this as a result of the requirement to starve prior to surgery. If in doubt, contact your Eye Unit.

Food and drink

If you are having a local anaesthetic, most units will be happy for you to eat and drink beforehand, but it is not sensible to have an enormous meal just before the operation. Drink fluids normally, but remember that if you want to pass urine, this is best done before the operation begins! Do not drink any alcohol before your surgery, although a glass of wine or beer when you return home is not unreasonable – as long as you have not had a general anaesthetic or sedation.

Patients having a general anaesthetic need to starve beforehand. This usually involves no food for six hours, and no fluids for four hours before the operation, although some anaesthetists will allow small volumes of water (approximately 100ml) up to two hours before the operation. Again, it is important to follow the specific instructions given. Sadly, some people fail to do this, and the surgery may have to be postponed.

Try to stay calm. It is natural to feel a little anxious, and the staff involved with your care will be used to dealing with people who feel worried. However, the operation is not the ordeal that many people envisage and – strange as it may seem – I regularly have patients who comment that they actually quite enjoyed the day! You may not feel quite as enthusiastic as this, but preparation is the key to being as calm as possible. Fear of the unknown is what is most daunting, and having read this book and any information that your local unit has provided will prepare you well in this regard. In the next chapter we shall consider what actually happens during the operation, including some of the more technical aspects of what the surgeon does.

6

The operation

Cataract surgery is usually undertaken with the patient lying back on a couch, the head steadied in a hollow of a firm pillow. This makes it easier to keep still, and assists the surgeon in positioning your head. Before starting the operation, you will be helped on to the couch, and placed in position. If you are very uncomfortable, it is best to mention this now, rather than once the operation has started.

It is routine to undertake some kind of monitoring of the pulse and sometimes take blood pressure or an ECG during surgery. To this end, you may have a little clip placed on your finger to monitor your pulse, and possibly sticky electrode pads put on your chest if an ECG is required. A blood pressure cuff may be placed on your arm, which inflates and squeezes the arm periodically to check the blood pressure. In addition, sometimes a small plastic cannula is placed into a vein in your wrist, in order to give you any drugs during the operation should these be necessary. This is an extra safety measure, and is not routinely undertaken in all units.

Following administration of the anaesthetic, a drape is placed over the face to keep hair and lashes out of the operating field. This is usually a type of paper towel, with a window of sticky plastic covering the eye. It is placed in position after cleansing of the skin with an antiseptic solution. The drape covers the other eye, but the surgeon has access to the eye to be operated on through a small hole that he cuts in the drape. A support is then placed in position to help keep the eyelids open. This means that you do not have to worry about blinking during the procedure. Once the drape is in position, it is lifted off your mouth, so

41

that it is not covered. If you are having only drops as an anaesthetic, you will be able to see what is going on up until this point, although not once the operation starts. As the surgeon switches on the microscope light, there is an intense brightness, following which there is no vision in the eye, although often a sensation of coloured lights.

The sensations experienced during the procedure depend upon the type of anaesthetic used. Obviously with general anaesthesia, the patient is aware of nothing. With a local anaesthetic, either of the sort given by needle or of the sub-tenon type discussed earlier, there is usually no sensation, other than sometimes an awareness that something is going on, rather as a tooth may feel that has been numbed by the dentist. With drops alone, there is often a slight feeling of pressure, and more awareness of bright, coloured shapes. Neither of these is unpleasant. Pain is not normal, and in the unlikely event that you experience pain with any form of anaesthetic, you should draw this to the surgeon's attention.

Many surgeons are happy to allow patients to speak directly to them while they operate, although they may request that you keep quiet at certain delicate stages, since sometimes talking can move the eye a little. I find that many people are more relaxed if they talk to me as I operate, and I enjoy many conversations with them during surgery. Other surgeons prefer silence. It is usual for somebody to hold the hand of a patient having a local anaesthetic, and they may ask that you squeeze their hand if you wish to speak, so that some sudden movement does not surprise the surgeon. Often background music is played to overcome some of the variety of noises of monitors and machines in the operating theatre.

How is cataract surgery undertaken?

You may not be interested in the technical details of how surgery is performed, and it is not necessary to read this section unless you are, since all the details of what you will experience are described elsewhere. However, for those who wish to know more, this section may be of interest.

The incision

In order to remove the lens and replace it with another, it is necessary to make a small incision in the eye placed either under the upper lid, or at the outer side of the cornea between the upper and lower lids. It is placed just at the junction between the clear cornea, and the white of the eye, and is constructed such that it is self-sealing. This is done by creating a sort of flap within the tissues of the eye, so that it is usually not necessary to place a suture to close it. It is 2.8mm in width, this being the size required by most modern ultrasound probes. In addition, a smaller incision is placed a little further around the junction of the cornea and the white of the eye, through which the surgeon can introduce a second instrument to aid with the surgery.

Once the incision has been completed, a sticky, clear gel is introduced into the eye, which allows it to stay formed. Without it, the fluid contained in the eye would just gush out, and leave the eye soft.

Opening the lens bag

The goal of surgery is to remove the lens from its natural bag, leaving the bag sufficiently intact to support the new lens. It is rather like removing the chocolate from the inside of a sugar-coated chocolate sweet, and replacing it with new chocolate, but leaving a hole in the front of the sugar coating. The first step in achieving this is to make a circular tear in the front of the bag, and this is done with a fine instrument like a bent needle. Although the front of the bag is extremely thin (approximately 20 microns), it is relatively strong, as long as the circular tear that is made in it is continuous, rather than a series of cuts similar to the perforations around a postage stamp. Ideally the circle of the front of the bag that is removed should be about 6mm in diameter. This leaves sufficient rim of the front of the bag to support the new lens, but allows adequate access to the interior of the bag to remove the old lens and insert the new one. To assist the lens removal, water is then injected between the bag and the lens to separate the two, and allow the lens to move freely within the bag. This is the equivalent of injecting in between the chocolate and sugar of the sweet, in order to separate them.

Phacoemulsification

This is a long word to explain a simple concept! *Phaco* derives from the Greek, meaning lens, and *emulsification* is exactly what it says – turning into an emulsion. *Phacoemulsification* therefore is simply the process whereby the lens is turned into a fluid that can be sucked out of the eye. The key to this process is the ultrasound probe. This consists of a hand-held instrument, similar in size to a rather fat pen, which contains within it an ultrasound crystal. When electrically activated, it causes vibration at ultrasonic frequency of a hollow needle, which in turn leads to the production of an acoustic sound wave just ahead of the needle tip, which is inserted into the eye. The products of the liquefied lens are sucked up through the centre of the hollow needle and removed from the eye. The power of the system is controlled by the surgeon through a foot pedal.

Around the needle tip is a sleeve, and there is a continuous irrigation of sterile fluid between the two. This ensures not only that the eye does not collapse as material is sucked from it, but also that there is adequate cooling of the needle by the irrigating fluid to prevent it heating up and burning the eye. The flow of fluid and power of suction from the eye through the needle are also controllable.

Using this instrument, the surgeon is able literally to

sculpt the lens within its bag, taking care, of course, not to damage the bag itself. Although there are many different strategies for the removal of the lens, the basic principle of all of them is to break the lens into several fragments (often four quadrants) and then use the ultrasound probe to emulsify and suck up these segments. Most surgeons start the procedure by creating grooves in the lens with the machine first, which then allows it to be cracked into several segments. Others prefer to 'chop' the lens into pieces using a small blade introduced through the second, smaller incision.

Once this has been completed, there is always some residual lens material still stuck to the inside of the bag, and this is removed with another instrument, which sucks up the material, at the same time as the eye is kept formed by infusion of fluid. This is in many ways similar to the phacoemulsification probe, but without the ultrasound component. Only when the lens bag is pristine can the new lens be inserted.

The new lens

Modern lenses are made from a variety of materials, including high-grade Perspex, silicone and acrylics. Increasingly, there is a tendency to use lenses that can be folded, so that they can be introduced into the eye without further enlargement of the wound. This avoids creating extra distortion or *astigmatism*, and also obviates the need for sutures in most cases.

There are various ingenious techniques for folding lenses, and many are now inserted using an introducer, which injects the lens into the bag. Apart from the central optical portion of the lens, there are two flexible, expanding loops extending from the lens, which gently spring out into the lens bag. It is these that keep the lens stable. A diagram of a modern lens implant is shown in Figure 2.

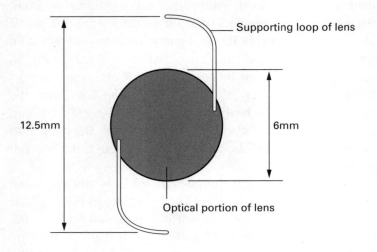

Figure 2

I was once operating on a lady while explaining, at her own request, the procedure to her and an observing surgeon. When it came to the point of inserting the new lens, I explained '. . . and now you will see that I am introducing the new lens into the old bag'.

'Who are you calling an old bag?' she exclaimed. I realized to my horror what I had said, and apologized profusely. Luckily she saw the funny side of the situation! This embarrassing – but true – story illustrates that although the lens that is inserted is perfect, and remains so indefinitely, it is indeed the patient's own original lens bag that supports it. This is important to realize in consideration of a situation that can arise some months after surgery whereby the bag itself can become cloudy. We shall consider this later in the next chapter. The other significance of the bag is that if it is either inherently weak, or is damaged by the surgery, it may not be sufficiently strong to support the new lens. Although this is a rare occurrence, it is one that can even prevent lens implantation in some cases.

Final checks

Once the lens is safely in the bag, the operation is essentially finished. It is necessary to remove any residual gel that has been used to keep the eye formed, and also to check that there is no leak from the wound. The drapes are then removed from the face, and a protective plastic shield placed over the eye. This is usually transparent, and so, as vision recovers, the eye is able to see a little. Once any attached monitors have been removed, the patient is then guided off the couch. Operation complete.

7

After the operation

The sensations immediately after surgery are variable, dependent not least upon the type of anaesthetic that has been used. Patients who have had a local anaesthetic injection, either using a needle or by the sub-tenon technique, may well find that the upper lid is closed at the end of surgery. This is because it is often paralysed by the local anaesthetic, and can take some hours to fully recover. In addition, the muscles that move the eye take time to recover their normal movement, and double vision is common while this is occurring. If the upper lid is closed, then this will mask the double vision until it opens.

Whatever the form of anaesthetic used, the vision is usually very blurred immediately after surgery. This is for a number of reasons. First, the intense microscope light that is used during the operation bleaches the retina for some time, but also, the very large pupil confuses the image. If a local anaesthetic has been injected, it takes a while for its effect on the optic nerve to wear off, and there may be no vision at all until this occurs. Frequently, patients notice a red haze in front of the eye, which lasts for anything from a few hours up to several days, and this can occur under all forms of anaesthetic.

We shall discuss the matter of glasses in a later chapter, but it is important to realize that the strength of glasses needed after surgery is nearly always different to those worn beforehand. For this reason, the vision after surgery may not seem good until a change in glasses has been made. Do not go to your optometrist for this until you are advised, however.

Pain is not usual after cataract surgery, but as the local

49

anaesthetic wears off it is not unusual to experience some mild discomfort. This tends to be noticeable most when the eye moves, as the small wound in the eye rubs against the eyelid. If you are a little uncomfortable, two paracetamol tablets should be sufficient to relieve the discomfort, but any severe pain should be reported to the unit. Though rare, it is possible for pressure to build up during the first few hours after surgery, and this sometimes requires either tablets or removal of a small amount of fluid from the eye to relieve it.

The appearance of the eye, as opposed to the vision through it, is also variable in the earliest stages. Eyes that have had either form of local anaesthetic injection may appear somewhat swollen from this initially. Also, some blood in the white of the eye is not uncommon, but resolves spontaneously over a few days. This can also occur if an injection of antibiotic has been given at the end of the procedure. This practice is routinely undertaken by some units, and not by others. Do not be concerned therefore if you have these symptoms immediately following surgery. However, sudden swelling of the eyelids or the eyeball at any time later is *not* usual. So if you have this, you should make prompt contact with the unit, since it can – very rarely – indicate infection.

It is important to adhere strictly to the post-operative instructions issued to you by the unit in which you have surgery. There may be slight differences between these and the guidelines given below; if there are, you should adhere to those instructions issued by the local unit. Precise follow-up arrangements vary, both in timing and in the personnel undertaking them. You should be clear about what these are, however, before you leave the unit.

Some DO's and DON'T's

It is impossible to list every single activity that people undertake and give timings for when these things can be resumed. Common sense is the most valuable tool to guide you, but it is helpful to have some idea of what you can and can't do.

Probably the most important aspect of care for your eye in the first few weeks after surgery is the avoidance of infection. Great care is taken at the time of surgery to exclude any germs from the eye, and it is important to maintain high standards of hygiene, particularly during the first few weeks after the operation. Make sure that you always wash your hands before putting your drops in, and keep these drops in a safe, clean place. Avoid dirty environments where you might be at risk of contaminating the eye. This does not mean strict isolation at home, but it is not sensible to be digging the compost heap the day after surgery! If you go out in the wind, it may be sensible to wear some kind of protection such as glasses, to prevent particles blowing into the eye. Smoky, dusty atmospheres may well irritate the eye, even if no infection is caused.

Many people prefer to shower rather than take a bath these days. Although this is still acceptable immediately after your cataract operation, be sure that there is no high pressure of water entering the eye, and that you do not inadvertently get soap or shampoo in the eye, which may cause you to rub it without thinking. To this end, people with long hair are best advised to wash it with the head tilted back.

Modern surgery does not impose the restrictions that the larger wounds of days gone by did. In the past, patients were advised not to move suddenly, bend over or undertake any exercise for weeks after the operation. With a small, self-sealing wound, as used nowadays, these restrictions no

51

longer apply. I am quite happy for patients to resume normal activities as soon as they feel able, and was delighted that one of my patients won a bowls match the day after her surgery! Surprisingly, the tradition of not bending has been perpetuated by the medical and nursing professions, and many patients are still advised not to. As I have emphasized throughout this book, it is important to adhere to the local advice given, and if you are advised to restrict activities in any way, it is sensible to follow this advice. There may be particular reasons that it has been given, which you should respect.

Swimming is a wonderful way to keep fit, which many people enjoy. One of the few restrictions I impose on my patients is that if they swim, they should not dive underwater for several weeks, in order to avoid the increased pressure exerted by the water. Since all pools are now heavily treated with chemicals to kill germs, it is wise to wear goggles if you put your head underwater, simply to avoid the irritation such chemicals cause, and the temptation to rub the eyes.

It is best not to plan to fly in an aircraft for at least two weeks after surgery, in order to avoid the pressure changes that occur on take-off and landing.

Normal, gentle exercise is perfectly acceptable, even more vigorous fitness training in the gym can be resumed after a week.

The question of driving after surgery is sometimes a difficult one to answer. The legal standard for driving in the United Kingdom is the ability to read a number plate at 20.5 metres, and it does not matter if this is with just one eye, or both, as long as the field of vision is good. Many patients will easily achieve this immediately after surgery, either with the operated eye, or with the fellow eye in which the vision is good. If the vision is satisfactory, it is therefore reasonable to drive on the day following surgery, as long as you are entirely confident about your vision. It is important to remember that you should not drive within 24 hours of a general anaesthetic. Many patients do not feel confident enough to drive until they obtain new glasses, which may be about six weeks after surgery. Bear in mind that the point of focus will have been changed by the surgery, and it is quite possible that the two eyes will not be in balance, at least for a while after. *If in doubt, do not drive.*

Complications in cataract surgery are rare, and if all went well at the time of the operation it is very unusual for anything serious to develop afterwards. There are exceptional events that can occur, however, which require early treatment. Although you should not sit worrying about whether these might happen, it is useful to have some knowledge about some of them, so that you can seek help if it should be needed. Do not be worried about false alarms. If you have *any* doubts at all about your eye after the operation, you should get in touch with the Eye Unit. Failing this, if you are unable to contact them for any reason – if, for example, you are somewhere else staying with friends – then attend an Accident and Emergency department. It is essential to seek help if something seems to be going wrong, even if it is only for reassurance that it is not.

In the next chapter, we shall consider some of the complications of cataract surgery in detail.

8
Complications

There is no operation without any risk at all of possible complications, and it is important to consider the likelihood and consequences of these, before even making a decision to undertake, or undergo, surgery in the first place. We have talked about weighing the risks and benefits of an operation earlier in the book, but clearly any meaningful consideration of these requires some understanding of possible complications.

If a complication does occur, it is important that it is dealt with in an appropriate and timely manner. From the patient's point of view, this means making early contact if something appears not to be right. This may take the form of an unexpected event, such as sudden loss of vision or onset of severe pain, or simply a deviation from what you were expecting. Inevitably this means some false alarms, and you should not be worried or embarrassed about these. It is much better to seek help if there is any concern than to miss the opportunity for early treatment should it prove necessary.

Complications do not necessarily occur through anybody doing anything wrong, and unfortunately are often just events that occur in spite of proper treatment. Certainly it is possible for human error to contribute, and this may be on the part of the surgeon, anaesthetist, or anybody else involved in treatment (including, sometimes, the patient!). If this is the case, an honest discussion about what has happened is best, and we shall consider this later in the book.

It is not helpful to list in great technical detail every possible adverse event that can occur, but there are a number of potential complications that we should consider

55

here. The risks of these are often difficult to predict, since some are so infrequent that figures become a little meaningless; and others may be rare in the general population, but more likely in patients with a particular predisposition. For example, permanent cloudiness of the cornea after surgery is very uncommon, but if it does occur, it almost always does so in patients with an inherently weak cornea, which may be identifiable before surgery. If you are at risk of a particular complication such as this, it should be highlighted in the discussions before your operation.

It can be difficult to interpret the rate of complications, which vary in degree of seriousness, because if a complication does occur, it is naturally always very serious for the individual concerned. It is still useful, though, to have some idea of the incidence of the more serious events, and I have tried to do this below.

Complications that can occur

1 Rupture of the lens bag

The usual intention in cataract surgery is to remove the cataract lens from the bag within the eye in which it is situated, and to replace it with an implant, which is put in the bag in the same position as the natural lens was. The bag is extremely thin (around 20 microns) and delicate, and in some patients it can rupture during the course of the surgery, making it difficult to implant the lens. Usually it is still possible to implant a new lens, securing it in a slightly different way. Sometimes rupture of the bag leads to loss of some of the vitreous gel behind the bag. This in itself is replaced naturally, but it is important for the surgeon to undertake further surgery (at the time of the operation) to clear this gel away. Very rarely, it is necessary to undertake further surgery on a separate occasion in order to achieve this, and even sometimes delay implantation of the new lens. This complication is more likely in patients whose lens bag is very weak to start with, which includes those who are very short-sighted or who have particular types of glaucoma. Overall, the incidence reported is about 3 per cent. The majority of eyes in which it occurs will still recover good vision.

2 Dropped nucleus

The nucleus is the central part of the lens, which in a cataract may comprise the bulk of it. The aim of surgery is to remove this from the eye, but rarely (in about 1 in 300 patients) some, or all, of the nucleus may fall back into the vitreous gel. This can only occur if either the lens bag or the fine filaments attaching it to the eye are broken. Again, this is more common in those who are extremely short-sighted or those with a particular form of glaucoma. The situation is more serious than simple rupture of the lens bag, since if left in the eye, the now dislocated lens causes intense inflammation and raised pressure. It is therefore necessary for the lens to be retrieved from the back of the eye, often involving another operation which is usually done under general anaesthetic by a specialist experienced in retinal surgery.

Again, the outcome is usually good, but recovery is more prolonged, and the risks of retinal detachment or other damage to the vision are increased.

3 Corneal oedema

Oedema means water logging, and *corneal oedema* means swelling of the cornea with water, such that it becomes opaque. Sometimes there is a transient swelling of the cornea after surgery, which settles spontaneously, particularly if the pressure in the eye rises in the few hours after operation. If this develops, the surgeon may either give medication to lower the pressure, or just allow a little of the excess fluid in the eye out, by gently touching the side of the wound. This is painless and leads to rapid resolution of the problem. Sometimes, however, swelling of the cornea after surgery is permanent, if the inner lining of the eye – called the *endothelium* – is weak. There are situations in which this weakness can be predicted before surgery, and although this does not necessarily imply that the cornea will become cloudy afterwards, the risk of it needs consideration. Unfortunately, it is also possible for a cornea that looked quite healthy before the operation to swell in this way. If it fails to clear, and it can take some weeks to do so, then it may even be necessary to replace the cornea with a transplant.

4 Endophthalmitis

This term refers to infection within the eye, and is one of the complications most feared by eye surgeons, since potentially it can lead to total loss of vision in the eye. It is rare, occurring in approximately 1 in 1,000 cataract operations and, if treated promptly, sight can usually be restored – if not to normal, at least to something useful. The condition usually develops between two and ten days after surgery, and should be suspected if there is either a sudden drop in vision or onset of pain. Often there is associated swelling of the eyelids and redness of the eye. Treatment involves an urgent operation to take samples from the eye to identify any germs present, and injection of very powerful antibiotics into the eye. It can sometimes be difficult to distinguish endophthalmitis from a more vigorous than normal inflammation in the eye, but when in doubt a surgeon will always assume there is some infection, since if the opportunity to treat it is missed, it is likely that the vision will be lost.

5 Retinal detachment

The risks of retinal detachment with modern surgery are small, affecting approximately 1 in 200 eyes. Rupture of the lens bag increases the risk, and very short-sighted individuals are also more at risk of retinal detachment. The symptoms of retinal detachment are often of flashing lights, followed by the appearance of a curtain over part or all of the field of vision. If this does occur, surgery is necessary to fix the retina back in place. Although this is not always successful, results from modern retinal surgery are usually good. Once again, early diagnosis is important, since this very much improves the chances of good final vision, and it is important to seek early attention should these symptoms develop.

6 Wound problems

The wounds used in modern surgery usually do not require suturing, but there are circumstances under which it may be preferable to place a stitch. These include the possibility of leakage from the wound, which, although rare, can occur either if the tissues are poor, or if they have been overheated by the ultrasound probe. This can occur in particularly dense cataracts, although the surgeon should take precautions to minimize the likelihood of this. If a wound is found to be leaking after the operation is complete, it may even be necessary to place a suture at a second operation. Thankfully, this complication is rare now that modern instruments and techniques have evolved to minimize its occurrence.

It is not uncommon to be able to feel the wound in the first few days or even weeks after surgery. This is most noticeable when the eye moves, or if the eye is inadvertently touched. The cornea heals very slowly, but since the wound seals itself even before the tissues have healed over, this is not a problem.

Modern surgery causes very little distortion of the

cornea, and therefore the amount of *astigmatism* caused is minimal or none. Sometimes such distortion may be unintentionally caused by the operation, or a surgeon may even deliberately position or construct the wound differently to try and neutralize distortion that existed before the surgery. In either situation, the vision is not immediately stable after the operation, and may take some weeks to become so.

7 Refractive surprise

The *refraction* of the eye is the measure of its point of focus, and we have seen earlier how, within limits, this can be controlled by selection of the lens implant. Although generally the predictions made by calculations based on the biometry (measurements of the eye undertaken before surgery) are quite accurate, there can be unexpected results. These are often termed a *refractive surprise*. Such an error may be a result of inaccurate measurements of the eye, or of mislabelling of a lens implant, or through the formula used to calculate the lens power simply not working for that eye. The increasing accuracy of measurements and the availability of a variety of formulae, which can be used for different sizes of eye, have seen a reduction in the number and magnitude of errors of lens implantation. It is therefore unusual to have to undertake further surgery to correct such surprise results, but in exceptional circumstances, this may be the only option. Once a lens implant is in place, it is not readily removed, and although surgery, if necessary, can be undertaken to remove the lens and replace it, it is also possible to implant another lens on top of the one of the wrong power. An alternative is the use of laser surgery to the cornea, but this would not be undertaken until the eye had fully settled from the cataract operation.

The point of focus for the eye is not immediately fixed after the surgery, and minor changes in the lens position, which occur in the initial days after operation, change the refraction. It is for this reason that glasses are not prescribed until a few weeks after surgery. Equally, although gross errors of lens power may be apparent immediately, what may seem wrong straight after surgery may turn out to be fine once the eye has settled, and vice versa.

8 Thickening of the lens bag

Once the natural lens of the eye has been replaced with a plastic one, the back of the lens bag can develop some thickening, and consequently lead to blurring of vision. This can occur in up to 10 per cent of patients undergoing surgery, although in many the visual effects are only slight. It occurs usually a year or so after the operation, and is caused by the backward growth of cells from the rim of the front of the bag. Strangely, the thickening may occur in one eye of a patient, and not in the other, even though both eyes apparently underwent identical surgery. Although there are various theories as to why it may or may not occur, there is still much that remains unknown about its causation. There is good evidence that certain lens materials are more prone to causing such thickening of the bag than others, and the shape and size of the lens implant may also play a part. Whether such a common development, which occurs so long after routine surgery, should be called a complication is arguable. Certainly, it is not anybody's fault, but in practical terms, if it is causing visual difficulties, it may require treatment. Thankfully, this is easily undertaken as an outpatient, using laser to make a small hole in the bag, and takes only a few minutes. There is very little risk to such treatment, although it is possible for either the lens implant to be damaged by the laser, or occasionally for the retina to be damaged.

Unfulfilled expectations

It is important to distinguish complications from side effects and unfulfilled expectations. This may sound a rather semantic argument, but there is a significant difference. It is a common side effect of cataract surgery using a local anaesthetic injection, for example, to have blurred or double vision immediately afterwards, which lasts for some hours. It is not a complication, whereas blurred vision after the operation because of swelling of the cornea most certainly is. The failure of vision to recover to 6/6 after a routine operation, because there is some other disease within the eye – such as macular degeneration – is again not a complication, since the surgery has in no way caused it. It may, however, lead to unfulfilled expectations if the patient had anticipated full recovery to 6/6, which was not achieved.

These examples illustrate two important principles. The first is that if a particular side effect, which is entirely predictable, is going to cause sufficient upset as to put you off surgery, then it is obviously best not to proceed, rather than be distressed when it occurs. Few people will be so disturbed by the thought of a few hours of double vision as to not want to go ahead with the operation, but it may be a reason to choose a different form of anaesthesia. The second principle is that it is important, as much as possible, to have an idea of what outcome to expect. In the above example, for instance, if the macular degeneration had been diagnosed before the surgery, and the patient given an appropriately cautious prognosis, he would have been able to make an informed decision as to whether to have the operation. Hopefully, he would not have been surprised if he then failed to achieve 6/6 vision, and we have already seen that significant improvements in vision can be made, even when the goal of 6/6 is unachievable.

More case histories

We'll conclude this chapter with case histories of patients who have suffered various complications, with varying outcomes. None of these stories represents an inevitable outcome from the particular complication discussed, as of course the final result depends not only on the nature of the problem, but also on the speed and effectiveness of treatment, and the inherent strength of the eye.

Alfred

Alfred had cataract surgery to his right eye when he was 67. For some years before the operation his vision had been poor, and was gradually deteriorating. He had given up driving six months previously, and was finding it hard to read. His surgery was straightforward. He had drops alone for the anaesthetic, which he found quite comfortable.

On waking the day after the operation, he was astounded by the improvement in his vision. Colours seemed so vivid, and he could see birds at the bottom of his garden. His eye felt comfortable, but on the morning of the third day after surgery it began to ache a little. By the evening it had become quite painful, and he noticed that his vision was a little blurred. He woke up in the night because his eye was so sore, and by the next morning he was horrified when he realized that he could only see shapes through it, and all the clear detail had gone. His wife noticed that by this time the eye looked red, and the lids were swollen.

He telephoned the Eye Unit, and was told to come in immediately for assessment, and it was there that a diagnosis of infection within the eye was made (endophthalmitis). Within two hours he found himself in the operating theatre again, where they injected antibiotics inside the eye, after samples had been taken from it.

Alfred needed to stay in hospital for six days, and it took several weeks before his vision recovered to any degree. Even when the eye had finally settled, and he had new glasses, it never recovered to the level he had experienced the day after surgery.

This case is an example of one of the most serious of complications that can occur, and there are several lessons to learn from it. Although endophthalmitis is very rare, it is important to be aware of its symptoms, since early treatment is critical. A delay of even 24 hours can mean the difference between recovery to near normal vision, and total blindness in the eye. Alfred first noted symptoms of pain on the morning of the third day after surgery, but did not seek help until a day after that. Although he was still in time to save the eye, he might have had a better final outcome if he had contacted the Eye Unit or his GP earlier. This was not his fault, as he was simply trying not to trouble anybody, but it does show how necessary it is to get urgent treatment for this rare complication. It also demonstrates that it is important not to worry about 'false alarms' or feeling you are being a nuisance. You must also be clear who you need to contact if symptoms that worry you develop after the operation.

Brian

Brian had been told by his surgeon before his operation that it would be necessary to stretch his pupil in order to remove the lens, because it did not dilate properly when drops were instilled. He had a local anaesthetic, using an injection, which gave him complete comfort. Unfortunately, the surgeon had some difficulty removing the lens through the pupil, which, though it had been stretched, was still smaller than usual. As a consequence, the back of the lens bag broke, and although it was possible to remove all of the lens, there was insufficient support for a new lens. The surgeon had to make sure that the vitreous gel that came forward from the back of the eye was removed, and clear of the wound and the front chamber of the eye. He felt it unsafe to insert a lens at the time of the operation. Although Brian was aware that the surgery had taken longer than expected (about 40 minutes altogether), he had been comfortable throughout.

The surgeon explained to him afterwards what had happened, and that it would be necessary for him to have another operation to insert the lens at a later date. Brian was bitterly disappointed, particularly since the patient sitting next to him was telling everyone how well he could see, while Brian felt his vision was significantly worse than it had been before surgery.

Two months later, Brian underwent a second operation, again with a local anaesthetic, to insert the lens implant. He rapidly recovered full vision, and was thrilled with the final result. He decided to have the cataract in the other eye operated on also, and on this occasion everything went without a hitch. Although Brian had ultimately ended up with good vision in each eye, he still felt a little frustrated that it had taken two operations to get things right in the first eye.

Brian's eye sustained a rupture of the lens bag during surgery, probably as a result of the difficulties in operating through a small pupil. Although it is not uncommon for a pupil to widen up poorly, it is unusual for this to lead to complications. On this occasion it did, however, and the rupture was serious enough to prevent lens implantation. Sometimes, if the bag is torn just a little, it is still possible to place the lens in it, but once adequate support for a new lens has gone, the surgeon has to make a decision as to whether to use a different type of lens, which is placed in front of the iris, or to delay lens implant altogether until the eye has recovered from the operation.

There are various quite complex technical issues that influence this decision, including the chances of developing glaucoma, the shape of the eye, and any previous eye problems. If a lens implant is not inserted, the vision after is very poor until either a lens is inserted later, or until a contact lens is fitted, which can be used as an alternative to a lens implant. A lens actually within the eye is certainly more convenient than having to wear a contact lens, but if it is too risky to insert a lens even as a second procedure, or if the patient feels they really would not be prepared to have another operation, a contact lens will achieve the same effect.

Brian was quite brave in deciding to have the other eye operated on later. Before he chose to do so, he had a long discussion with the surgeon about the chances of a similar complication in this eye. He knew that he was slightly more at risk than most other patients, but all went well. Ultimately, he could not tell the difference between the vision in the two eyes.

Gladys

Gladys had her right cataract operated on when she was 77, and the left eye done 18 months later. Both operations seemed to go well, and she was pleased with the result. Approximately one year after surgery to the left eye, however, she noticed that the vision in the right was becoming blurred again. She had difficulty seeing in bright lights, and was unable to see the television at all clearly if she closed the left eye, which was now much stronger than the right. She wondered if she was developing cataract again in the right eye, although she seemed to remember somebody telling her this did not happen.

Gladys went to her own optometrist to check whether

her glasses needed changing. He told her that the bag supporting her lens had gone cloudy, and that she would probably need laser treatment for this. She was referred back to the Eye Unit, where the diagnosis was confirmed and she underwent laser treatment. This involved sitting at a machine very similar to the slit-lamp she had been examined at before, while the doctor placed a small lens on the front of her eye, which had been numbed with drops. She was asked to look straight ahead, and then for a few minutes was aware of intense bright flashes of light. The procedure was quite painless. She went home and was astonished that her vision had recovered to normal within about six hours. The left eye was never similarly affected, and both eyes still had very good vision four years later.

As we discussed before, this thickening of the lens bag, often termed *posterior capsule opacification*, is quite common. It is arguable whether to regard it as a complication, but it needs dealing with anyway. Many patients develop the change in one eye only, but others in both. Although typically the onset is one to two years after surgery, it can develop more quickly, and can even occur many years later. Treatment is usually quick and effective, and it rarely needs repeating.

In the rare cases of childhood cataract, when surgery may be undertaken even on babies, the development of thickening is much more common, and it is almost inevitable that treatment will be required at some stage. Furthermore, in children, such treatment may need repeating.

Attempts to minimize the chances of thickening of the lens bag have seen developments in the type of materials, design and shape of lens implants. In spite of these, it remains a common problem, but one that is usually readily dealt with.

*

Complications, of whatever nature, can be frightening, but it is important to realize that most of them can be resolved, leading to a good final outcome. In many cases, the degree of visual recovery depends upon early recognition of the problem and prompt management. Although the surgeon and his team should ensure that you, the patient, have ready access to advice when needed, it is important that you play your part by making contact whenever you have worries concerning the operation. The key throughout the process of cataract surgery is that both the patient and the Eye Unit are working together, and never is this more important than in the early recognition and treatment of complications.

9

The question of glasses

It seems that nothing confuses and concerns patients more after cataract surgery than the question of glasses. Part of the reason for this is that the situation is slightly different for almost everybody. One patient may have been very dependent on glasses before surgery, and find that he needs them less afterwards, while another may find that he wears them more than before, because he is suddenly able to read with them, which he was unable to do before the operation.

Understanding some principles

In order to understand such apparent inconsistencies, it is necessary to consider a few principles of how focusing is achieved by the eye, when viewing things at different distances. Again, it is helpful to think of the eye as a camera. The cornea and lens between them should focus an image clearly on the retina, just as a camera lens system focuses images on the film. In the normal sighted eye, images from the distance are brought sharply into focus on the retina, while the lens is in its 'relaxed' state. If we need to see objects closer than this, the lens needs to focus the rays of light more, and to do this it needs to make itself stronger. This it does by actually changing shape, and by becoming fatter, so bringing near objects into focus. This is illustrated in Figure 3.

As we get older, however, this ability of the lens to change focus is gradually lost. This is why we see people in their forties finding that they need to hold reading material at progressively further distances away to get it in focus, as the ability of the lens to change shape is lost. Eventually the

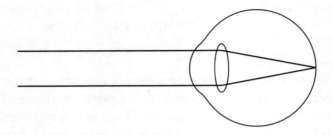

Rays of light from a distant object are almost parallel,
and are brought into focus by the lens in its relaxed state.

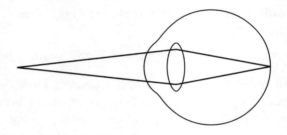

Rays of light from a near object are spreading out, and
so have to be focused more by the lens. It becomes fatter
to achieve this.

Figure 3

eye is only able to see distant objects in clear focus, at
which point the normal-sighted individual has to have
reading glasses.

This, then, is the situation for somebody who is normal-
sighted, but many of us are short- or long-sighted. What we
mean by these terms is that, if the eye is short-sighted, its
natural point of focus is not for the distance, but for near
objects. If such a person wishes to see clearly in the
distance, he needs to make his own natural lens weaker (the

opposite of what the normal-sighted person does to bring objects in focus for near vision). This he simply cannot do because although it is possible for the lens to become stronger by becoming fatter, it cannot become weaker. He therefore needs to wear glasses, which effectively 'weaken' the focusing power of his own lens.

The long-sighted person has his natural point of focus set not just in the distance, but beyond infinity. He may well be able to see in the distance by changing the shape of his natural lens to make it stronger, just as the normal-sighted person does to change from distance to near. However, to have to do this all the time for distance is tiring, and can cause double vision. If he is very long-sighted, his lens may not have sufficient power even when working at its strongest. He therefore needs glasses to 'strengthen' the focusing power of his own lens. Both short- and long-sighted individuals also suffer the same reduction in ability to change focus that the normal-sighted person does, of course.

Let us now consider how these principles relate to the situation after cataract surgery. It is possible, within certain limits of accuracy, to select the point of focus of an eye after surgery. This is done by calculating the power of lens implant to insert, from the measurements undertaken before surgery (biometry). The point of focus selected is fixed, and if focus is required at a different distance, it is necessary to wear glasses to achieve this. For example, if the eye is set for the distance, the vision for television, driving and other distance tasks may be good, without glasses, but reading glasses will be needed for near work. This situation is very similar to that of the normal-sighted individual we discussed above, once he has lost his ability to change focus at will, as happens around the age of 40 onwards. Since most patients having cataract surgery are older than this, and so have already lost this ability, they are not usually surprised or inconvenienced by this. Younger patients having cataract surgery, however, may well notice that they become more reliant on their glasses for reading, for example. Returning to the analogy of the camera, it is convenient to think of cataract surgery as replacing the lens, but with one of fixed focus.

Even this is something of an oversimplification. We all know of people who have had cataract surgery and claim never to have needed glasses again. This is certainly quite possible, either if one eye is set for a slightly different distance to the other, or if the patient is prepared to accept reasonable vision, rather than perfectly sharp vision. For example, somebody whose eye ends up in sharpest focus for objects viewed at 2 metres may still have sufficiently good distance vision for most activities, and yet be able to read reasonably small print. He may therefore decide not to wear glasses most of the time, and if the other eye is in focus for half a metre, he may never wear them at all. This sounds ideal, and for many patients it is, but if there is too great a disparity between the point of focus of the two eyes, they may not work well together, even if this is corrected with glasses. It is usual, therefore, to aim to reasonably match the focus of the two eyes. In addition, although the measurements and calculations involved in biometry are accurate and reliable, they cannot be guaranteed to be so precise in any individual as to be able to choose the point of focus absolutely.

Where will the eye be in focus after surgery?

We have seen that after surgery the eye will be set at a fixed focus, and that it is possible to choose where this point of focus will be, by selecting an appropriate power of lens implant. It is important to decide where the intended focus is to be, bearing in mind that even modern biometry has limits to its accuracy.

For most people, the choice for the point of focus would be the distance, so that they can see without glasses, and wear reading glasses for near vision only. There are circumstances, however, in which a different target of focus may be chosen, if for example the surgeon is trying to match the other eye. It is important to think about how the two eyes will work together, since if there is a large difference in focus between them, there will be confusion, and possibly even double vision.

Cataract surgery is a great opportunity to correct a high degree of short- or long-sight, but if only one eye is to be operated on, it is necessary to think about how the balance between the two eyes will be achieved, which we shall discuss shortly.

When is it possible to wear glasses again?

Once surgery is complete, and any anaesthetic has worn off, it is usual for there to be some vision almost immediately. This is often not clear, partly because of the bleaching of the retina caused by the bright microscope light, and partly because the pupil is usually still wide open for anything up to a few days after surgery, and this also interferes with focusing. In addition, changes to the focus occur over a period of a few days to several weeks, as the wound heals, and as the new lens settles into the lens bag. During this time, the bag can tighten up a little, and in so doing, slightly change the position of the lens in the eye, and hence its point of focus. For these reasons, it is usual not to prescribe glasses until a few weeks after surgery, when the situation can be expected to be stable. Even within a day or so, however, the new point of focus is reasonably stable in most cases.

Although it is wise not to buy new glasses immediately, it is perfectly reasonable to wear glasses as you wish, right from the time of the operation. These might be your old glasses, or even some borrowed ones if they help you to see better! If the eye has been set in focus for the distance, simple reading glasses available from the chemist may serve as a useful interim measure, pending a final spectacle prescription. Equally, if you find that you are now managing without glasses, this is perfectly acceptable. You will do yourself no harm by wearing glasses, or indeed not wearing glasses.

The final choice of glasses once all has settled depends not only on the new point of focus, but also on personal preference. Some patients are very keen to become less dependent on glasses after their surgery, and reduce or abandon spectacle wear, while others feel lost without them. In most cases, there is no reason not to resume wearing bifocal or multifocal lenses if this is your choice, or indeed even contact lenses if they are still necessary. It is best to discuss the type of glasses you want with your optometrist once you have been told you can go ahead with this by the Eye Unit.

If you are intending to have both eyes operated on for cataract, it is usual to wait until both operations have been done before buying new glasses. Obviously it is not sensible to have to have new glasses replaced *again*, just a few weeks after purchase, by having new ones made up after the first operation that will need replacing after the second eye has been operated on. Some people, though, who may find their vision difficult in this interim period, will choose to have new glasses made up after the first operation, knowing that the lens of the other side of the glasses will subsequently need replacing. If you intend to have the second eye operated on, it is sensible to make this clear to your optometrist when you visit.

Multifocal lenses

Multifocal lenses are lenses that offer a number of different points of focus. The concept is well established in glasses, the usual arrangement being a lens for the distance in the top segment of the glasses, one for seeing near objects at the bottom, and a transition zone in between, which provides focus in between distance and near.

There are also available multifocal lenses that can be implanted in the eye as the replacement lens for the cataract. Although these sound ideal, and theoretically might avoid the need for glasses altogether after surgery, they often do not provide quite the level of vision sought. This may be because of other limiting factors in the eye, such as astigmatism, or it may be because they can lead to dazzle and glare, with some loss of absolute clarity. In spite of continuing developments and improvements in lens design, so far the ideal of a perfect lens implant that can change focus at will with no optical aberrations has not been achieved.

Monovision

An alternative to a focusing lens is the concept of *monovision*. This refers to the situation whereby during surgery one eye is set in focus for near, and the other for distance. This can be an attractive, acceptable way out of glasses, and indeed accounts for the majority of patients who claim never to have needed glasses again after surgery.

Sometimes monovision may be achieved almost unintentionally, when surgery to the second eye brings the eyes into slightly different focus. Often a surgeon will intentionally choose to select a lens implant for the second eye that brings it into focus slightly nearer than the first, if the first is set for far distance, since we know that biometry is not absolutely accurate, and it is better to err on the side of bringing the second eye into focus *nearer* than the distance, rather than *beyond* it (in which case, of course, it would not be in focus anywhere, without glasses).

As a planned strategy, monovision is unfortunately variably tolerated. Although some patients relish the freedom of not wearing glasses, others find that they do not have full *stereovision*. If there is any biometry error, then having intentionally targeted to make the two eyes different, which is what monovision obviously implies, may prove to be unwise, and compound the error.

Astigmatism

We have made various references to *astigmatism* through this book, and now is an appropriate time to discuss the concept further. Astigmatism simply means distortion of the cornea, which in turn leads to distortion of the image formed. A useful analogy is to think of a cornea with astigmatism as looking like a rugby ball rather than a football. It is more curved in one direction than the other.

Astigmatism is not uncommon, and many of us have a small amount of corneal distortion without ever being aware of it. Greater degrees of distortion, however, require correction with glasses. One of the great advances in modern cataract surgery is that the small incisions used induce little or no astigmatism, whereas the larger wounds of the past routinely caused more distortion. It is even possible not only to avoid causing distortion, but to actually reduce the amount of *pre-existing* astigmatism by changing the placement of the surgical wound, or making additional partial thickness incisions in the cornea at specific locations. Although this can be helpful and appropriate in certain situations, it would be unrealistic to guarantee complete neutralization of astigmatism in all cases, and unexpected results can occur. If this sort of enhancement to the cataract surgery is contemplated, the surgeon should discuss your own specific situation with you.

Case histories

Because of the many varied situations in different individuals, it is not possible to give case histories of every possible outcome of surgery, but we will consider the results in two specific cases below:

Barbara again

Barbara was 72 when she underwent cataract surgery, and was already used to wearing glasses for reading. The surgeon selected a lens implant for her, which was intended to put the eye in focus for the distance. This worked well, and she found that she was able to see satisfactorily without glasses very soon after surgery. When she had her other eye operated on, a similar lens was inserted, which should have achieved the same point of focus. Again it was successful, and finally Barbara had new glasses just for reading. Although the two eyes were well matched, she was aware that the right eye was a little sharper for far distance vision, but that the left could manage rather better for objects somewhat closer.

This case history illustrates a very common situation, in that the two eyes ended up very slightly different in their point of focus, in spite of measurements and calculations suggesting that they both needed the same power of implant. The difference was so slight, though, that Barbara was only aware of it if she alternately covered one eye, and then the other, and the two eyes worked well together. Very few people have absolutely identical eyes, and it is not uncommon to find one ending up at a slightly different focus. In practical terms, this is not a problem.

Eric

Eric had been short-sighted since early childhood, and recalled wearing his first pair of glasses at the age of six. Since then he had needed progressively stronger lenses, and by the time of his cataract surgery he was wearing very thick-lensed spectacles.

His surgeon warned him that he would notice an imbalance between the two eyes after the operation, but that this could be addressed when he had the second eye operated on four weeks later. After the first operation, Eric was delighted to be able to see without his glasses, for the first time in years. He found that he was best in focus for the mid-distance, but that when he put his old glasses on, he could not see anything through the eye that had been operated on. During the four weeks before the second operation, he had some difficulty judging distances, and even managed to miss his cup when pouring from a teapot and so spilled tea on to the table. Once the second operation had been completed, Eric abandoned glasses altogether for distance vision, and just wore them for reading.

People who have been used to extreme short-sightedness for a long time love the independence from glasses that cataract surgery can offer them. Even if they are left a little short-sighted afterwards, and still wear glasses for distance, the benefit of not needing such thick, heavy glasses, with the restrictions they impose, is enormous. The period in between the two operations may be quite difficult, and the loss of stereovision is because the eyes are not able to join the two images now that they are so different. The lack of depth perception caused by this can result in accidents with a teapot (as in Eric's case) or, even worse, with a car. If you were still driving before cataract surgery in this sort of situation, it would be necessary to stop driving in the interim period between the two operations. Once the eyes are back in balance, following conclusion of surgery to the second eye, stereovision is recovered.

Conclusion of treatment

The final provision of glasses is usually the conclusion of the process of cataract surgery. As we have seen, although some people may not need glasses after their operation, most will find that they do (at least for some tasks), and it is important to have an assessment for glasses if you wish to achieve your best possible vision. Some people, so thrilled by the improvement achieved with surgery, omit the final step of having glasses fitted – and often to their detriment. It is a shame not to get the full benefit from surgery, and even if you subsequently choose not to wear glasses, it is worth seeing what improvement they would make by means of the final eye test. Such tests may be undertaken by an optometrist within the Eye Unit, or it may be suggested that your own optometrist do this. After all the work and planning, you should now be able to enjoy the benefits of improved vision.

10

Surgery on your second eye

Most of us have two eyes, and although cataract may only affect one of them, it is very common for the other eye also to be involved – even if to a lesser extent. So it is worth thinking about both eyes right from the earliest stages of planning cataract surgery, since it is important that they work together if possible. Such planning may involve not only consideration of how the two eyes will function together immediately after surgery, but also predicting how the vision in the eye that has not been operated on might change in the future.

Matching the eyes

We saw in the last chapter that the two eyes will not work together if there is a large difference in their focus, even when the vision is corrected with glasses. This is because the size of the image formed on the retina will be different in each eye, and the brain is unable to join the two to form a single, stereo image. Interestingly, if a contact lens is used rather than a spectacle lens, the image sizes are the same, and this can be a good way around such a problem of the eyes being out of balance. It is clearly preferable, however, to be able to see without the trouble of wearing contact lenses. To this end, it is usual to attempt to match the two eyes by appropriate selection of lens implant power at the time of surgery.

Often this is a simple process, but if there is pre-existing long- or short-sight that it is intended to correct at the time of the cataract surgery, thought needs to be given in advance as to how the eyes will manage to work together afterwards. If both eyes have cataract, then the solution is to match the two by operating on both of them and choosing the same point of focus for each, but if the second eye does not have a cataract, a decision has to be made as to where the focus should be. It is even possible to remove a natural lens that does *not* have cataract, in order either to match it to the other eye, or even just to cure short- or long-sightedness. This is termed *clear lens extraction*. Although this is a very effective technique for dealing with, in particular, high degrees of short-sightedness, we should not forget that cataract surgery is not without risk, and for this reason many surgeons feel unhappy about removing a clear, healthy lens.

When should the second eye be operated on?

If both eyes need cataract surgery, it may seem logical to operate on both at the same time, and since the operation is so quick, this is not a problem either for the patient or surgeon. There are, however, some rare complications in cataract surgery, which do not occur until a few days after the operation. In particular, the problem of endophthalmitis (which we discussed on page 58) can cause serious damage to the vision.

Although extremely unlikely, should this happen to both eyes, which were operated on at the same time, there could be a disastrous outcome of loss of vision in both. For this reason, many surgeons feel that surgery to both eyes at once is generally not wise.

Furthermore, it is often useful to know the outcome from surgery to the first eye before proceeding with the second. If the point of focus is different to that predicted, it is helpful to know this in order to make appropriate adjustments to the lens power selection for the second eye.

Different Eye Units will have different policies concerning how soon after the first operation surgery to the second eye can be undertaken. Generally, a period of at least several weeks is allowed to ensure that the first eye has fully settled.

Will surgery to the second eye be the same?

Assuming that surgery to the first eye went well, and that patient and surgeon were satisfied with the outcome, it is usual to proceed with the second eye in a similar manner, using the same type of anaesthetic, lens implant, and often the same surgeon.

If this was not the case, it is a time when consideration can be made to change, and you should speak out if you were not happy about the first operation. If, for example, you did not like the sensation of double vision after the local anaesthetic, to the extent that you felt this was not something you would wish to have again, it is an appropriate time to discuss this, and the various alternatives for the second eye.

Even if surgery is undertaken in exactly the same way, by the same surgeon, it is surprising to learn that very few patients perceive the two experiences as having been identical. Partly this is because it is difficult for a patient to remember the precise details of all that happened the first time, especially if they were slightly anxious, but also because the sensations experienced are often genuinely different. We discussed earlier how when using drops alone as anaesthetic there is usually the sensation of coloured lights during the surgery, and this may vary considerably between the two eyes. Local anaesthetic by injection or sub-tenon technique also varies in its effect. Sometimes there is no perception of light after the injection, while more commonly there is still some, but with variable visual sensation.

Immediately after the operation, the vision is usually blurred, but again the degree of blurring is often different between the two eyes; and even when the eye has settled, if you alternately cover one eye and then the other, there is often a difference in the point of focus between them.

What if I didn't get a perfect result with the first eye?

It can be a difficult decision as to what to do with the second eye if there has been a complication, or less than perfect result, with the first. On the one hand, there is the natural reluctance to expose the other eye to the same risks, but there is also potentially the opportunity to correct the vision by treating the second eye successfully. Obviously the matter needs some thought and discussion, and each individual will come to his own decision, with the support of those looking after him.

Perhaps the first consideration in such a decision is why the result was less than perfect. The surgery may have been uncomplicated, but the outcome poorer than hoped for because of an unrelated problem, such as macular degeneration, and in this situation it may well be that the same might happen in the other eye. We have already seen how difficult it can be to predict the outcome in such situations. If the result was not good because of a surgical complication, then it is worth trying to make an assessment of how likely this may be to occur to the other eye. Complications, by their very nature, are generally not predictable, but if an eye with an inherent weakness, such as a weak cornea, does not survive surgery, then it is more likely that the second eye may suffer a similar fate. This is not necessarily a reason not to operate on the second eye, but is certainly a reason to give the matter some further thought.

Other less than perfect outcomes may be easier to deal with. In particular, if there has been an unexpected biometry result, then it may well be possible to balance the two eyes by appropriate lens selection for the second eye. In this particular circumstance, it would be normal to repeat the measurements and establish whether there was any error in them.

In the rare event that surgery to the first eye led to complete blindness, it takes a degree of bravery on the part of the patient to have surgery to the now 'only' eye. The same considerations that we made earlier in the book about the risks and benefits need to be made, but obviously the very rare events that can lead to loss of vision need further serious consideration, as does the cause of failure in the first eye. Although both patients and surgeons prefer to have a 'back-up' eye, in the case of the worst happening, this is not always possible, and surgery to the only eye is not uncommon. The vast majority of these operations are routine with a good result, and generally people who have delayed having surgery to their second eye, because of problems with the first, wonder afterwards why they did not go ahead sooner. There is no absolute guidance to be given here, other than to advise that you should only go ahead once you feel ready.

11

Choices, choices

We live in an age of increasing choice, and though this is generally to our benefit, it can make life complicated if we are not prepared and informed sufficiently to make such choice. We have seen already that some aspects of cataract surgery require decisions to be made between the various options available. What sort of anaesthetic is best? What power of lens should be inserted? Should the other eye be operated on? These are all decisions that need to be made, and although they are not made by the patient in isolation, the more you understand the issues involved, the more you will be able to express your wishes and choose what is best for you. Having read this book so far, you should now be in a better position to do just this, and to discuss matters with the staff looking after you.

Not all units and surgeons offer precisely the same choices. Some may routinely use one form of local anaesthetic, and others may not have the option of general anaesthetic at all. Many surgeons still do not like to operate using drops alone as an anaesthetic, which from a technical point of view is somewhat more challenging. Equally there are different types of lens implant available, but generally any particular surgeon will use only a limited range of these, in order that he can provide consistent results, rather than switching from one to another. It is not a good idea to try and persuade a surgeon who is unfamiliar or unhappy with a particular technique into using it, and indeed he should not give in to such requests. If you feel strongly that you wish to have a particular type of lens, or anaesthetic, that he does not offer, then you should consider changing the surgeon you use rather than have him undertake something at which he is not expert. Similarly, a patient should not be forced to fit in with a system that does not accommodate his needs. There is sometimes a temptation to feel trapped within a process over which you have no control, but if you are not happy with the personnel and treatment planned for you, you should seek referral either to another surgeon within the unit, or another unit altogether. Hopefully, this should be a relatively rare situation, but confidence that all is being done for you in a manner with which you are happy is essential.

What are the choices in type of Eye Unit?

In recent years, there has been a huge expansion in the types of unit offering cataract surgery, both within the state and private sectors. Although the traditional eye department either within a large general hospital or standing alone still undertakes a large proportion of cataract surgery, there are other providers with different approaches. These include dedicated cataract units, often in purpose-built buildings, which undertake nothing but cataract operations, and mobile facilities of various types. The latter include large lorries, which tour the country with their own equipment and staff.

All of these units need to comply with certain standards to be allowed to continue in practice, but there are some practical differences between them that it is helpful to consider in choosing where you wish to have your surgery.

Let us consider some of the questions you should consider and be prepared to ask.

What do I need to know about the unit and staff?

Where will the surgery and the tests before and after the operation be undertaken?

This sounds an obvious question, but it is important that you are able to get to the unit for the tests such as biometry and any post-operative checks needed. These may all be undertaken in the same unit, but could be in different places.

Who will be looking after me?

Again, this is fundamental to confidence in the process. Most probably there will be a number of people looking after you, including nurses, optometrists, surgeons and others. In some units you may be assessed by one doctor, and operated on by another, whom you do not meet until the day of the surgery, or in some cases do not meet at all, other than as you lie on the couch to be operated on. This may sound somewhat impersonal, and is thought of by some as 'conveyor belt' surgery, but if the surgery is of the highest standard, and you have other carers such as nurses whom you have met before, who help you through the operation, you may not feel the need to make personal acquaintance with the surgeon. After all, very few of us meet the captain of the aircraft we board! Other people, however, do not like the idea of not meeting their surgeon, and prefer to have some kind of personal rapport with him. It is not unreasonable to ask the simple question 'Who will be doing my operation?' and to expect an honest reply, including any statement of whether any trainee doctor will be involved in your surgery. Rest assured that if this is the case, he will have been thoroughly assessed first, and only allowed to operate within his own capabilities.

Whom do I contact if I am worried?

We have seen earlier the importance of making early contact at any stage, whether this be before or after the operation, if you are worried. In Chapter 8, the dangers of delay were highlighted, and it is therefore essential that you are clear how to get in touch if there is any suspicion of a problem. This means a phone number or place of contact 24 hours a day, seven days a week. Emergencies do not just happen in office hours! It is helpful also to know where you might be expected to report to if you need to attend with an emergency. If your surgery was undertaken in a mobile unit, for example, it may have moved by the time you have a problem, and it is vital to know where to turn to.

Does the unit offer the service I want?

Obviously any cataract unit will be able to offer cataract surgery, but there are some specific requirements of certain patients that may need consideration. For example, a patient wishing to have a general anaesthetic is unlikely to be able to have this done in either a mobile or 'ambulatory' (walk-in and walk-out) cataract unit, which caters for surgery only using local anaesthetic. It is not practicable for such units to be able to offer facilities for general anaesthetic, and you are likely to need to go to a more conventional hospital if you need this.

Some patients may need to spend a night either in hospital, or at least under some supervision after their operation. Once again, this applies principally to those having a general anaesthetic, and since they comprise a small minority of patients having cataract surgery, facilities may not be available for this in all units.

How do I assess the unit?

It is vital to have confidence in the people treating you, and there are ways of acquiring information about them.

Although league tables of performance are very fashionable in all walks of life now, there are few published indices of outcomes which directly compare surgical results between different units and surgeons. At the time of writing, there are none available for cataract surgery in the United Kingdom, and even should they become so in the future, they would need interpreting with caution. A unit that may have a larger population of, for example, diabetics, or in which there is a surgeon accepting referrals from other specialists of particularly complex cases, may not appear as good on paper as a unit taking only selected cases.

What should be available, however, are results of audit within a unit. Cataract surgery is very amenable to analysis, since many parameters of success or failure are readily measured. For example, it should be possible for a unit to provide figures of the incidence of the major complications discussed earlier, such as posterior capsule rupture, dropped nucleus and endophthalmitis, together with a measure of the accuracy of the biometry. But even with this information, it can be difficult to assess the unit purely on the basis of figures; however, if you are interested and request this data, then it should be available. If it is not, or is refused, then you may be right to wonder why.

Word of mouth remains a useful, though not infallible, source of information. If you know a number of friends who have had positive experiences in a particular unit or with a particular surgeon, then this is encouraging. It is, of course, no guarantee that you will enjoy the same, but is a good start. Your GP may be able to advise you about referral, and be aware of the various advantages and drawbacks to the different services on offer, as may your optometrist.

Perhaps most important of all is the feeling you yourself have about whether the unit you are referred to will suit your needs. There are different sorts of service provision, and different sorts of patients. You should be happy that you have the information you need, the rapport with staff, and the facility to ask questions and get in touch without a problem. If this is not the case, then it is better to change to somewhere that you are happy with, rather than go ahead without confidence, and regret this later.

In general . . .

Most patients have a very happy experience with modern cataract surgery, and are keen to have the other eye operated on, and recommend the operation to others. Things certainly have moved on from the surgery we described in the Introduction, and you can expect a much more comfortable and successful experience than did the patients of 20 years ago. I hope that with the knowledge you have acquired in this book, you will be able to proceed with confidence and optimism towards a successful outcome.

12
Further information

The aim of this book has been to provide all of the information that you need to understand about cataract and its treatment. It should not be necessary to undertake further research, but some readers may be interested in the more technical aspects of surgery, or the new developments constantly being pioneered. These principally involve modifications to surgical techniques and lens implants, as new materials and technologies evolve. The nature of such advances is that they are generally reported in the medical press, which can be somewhat complex and full of jargon.

Because of the rapid changes occurring in this field, books may be unable to keep up with the very latest advances, and keeping in touch with the very latest technology often involves reading journals or doing research on the internet. Do not, though, be concerned if you are not completely conversant with the most recent advances: it is your specialist's job to ensure that he or she is, and to make you aware of any relevant changes in practice.

Listed below are some suggestions for further reading. The internet provides an enormous resource of further information, and the websites listed should provide current and useful knowledge and opinion.

Further reading and websites

Books and journals
Desai, P., Minassian, D. C., and Reddy, A., 'National cataract surgery survey 1997–8: a report of the results of

the clinical outcomes', *British Journal of Ophthalmology*, 1999, 83 (12), pp. 1336–40.

Eke, T., Thompson, T., and Thompson, J. R., 'The national survey of local anaesthesia for ocular surgery', *Eye*, 1999, 13, pp. 189–204.

Kanski, J., *Clinical Ophthalmology*. Butterworth Heinemann, 2003.

Leaming, D. V., 'Practice styles and preferences of ASCRS members – 2003 survey', *Journal of Cataract and Refractory Surgery*, 2004, 30, pp. 892–900.

NHS Executive, *Action on Cataract – Good Practice Guidance*. February 2000.

Reidy, A., *et al.*, 'Prevalence of serious eye disease and visual impairment in a north London population: population-based, cross-sectional study', *British Medical Journal*, 1998, 316, pp. 1643–6.

Websites

www.rcophth.ac.uk

The website of the Royal College of Ophthalmologists provides much useful information, including the downloadable patient information booklet 'Understanding Cataracts', produced jointly with the Royal National Institute for the Blind. It also offers some glimpses into the organization of training for surgeons in the United Kingdom.

www.nurseseyesite.nhs.uk

This website was set up and is run by a group of specialist eye nurses. Although it is principally a forum for discussion and education between nurses, it also contains much useful patient information about cataract and other eye diseases.

www.rnib.org
This is the website of the Royal National Institute for the Blind, and it offers much help and advice to all eye patients, whether they are blind, or simply seeking extra information. There is a useful database of hospital resources within the United Kingdom.

www.healthyeyes.org.uk
This website is also run by the Royal National Institute for the Blind, and contains useful information about eyesight, including many relevant pictures and illustrations.

www.mrcophth.com/Historyofophthalmology/cataract
This website gives a good account of the history of cataract and its treatment. Although much is not relevant to modern practice, it is a fascinating insight into the evolution of surgery for cataract.

www.sightsavers.org
This website details some of the marvellous work undertaken by Sight Savers, a charity that performs approximately 175,000 cataract operations a year. In addition, there is much useful information about cataract and its treatment.

www.moorfields.org.uk
This is the website of Moorfields Eye Hospital. It contains much general information about many eye diseases, including cataract, and has numerous helpful diagrams and illustrations. There is a good section on Frequently Asked Questions.

Index